T0246209

GOOD NATURE

*Why Seeing, Smelling, Hearing,
and Touching Plants is
Good for Our Health*

KATHERINE WILLIS

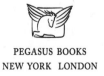

PEGASUS BOOKS
NEW YORK LONDON

GOOD NATURE

Pegasus Books, Ltd.
148 West 37th Street, 13th Floor
New York, NY 10018

ISBN: 978-1-63936-764-1

10 9 8 7 6 5 4 3 2

Printed in the United States of America
Distributed by Simon & Schuster
www.pegasusbooks.com

Contents

Introduction

I originally trained as a palaeoecologist.

That's a statement that can stop the conversation dead at parties, since not many people know what it is (never mind how to spell it).

Actually, it's a fascinating branch of science that uses the fossilised remains of plants to reconstruct vegetation changes over time in response to climate change, human impact and other environmental drivers. The results provide important scientific knowledge, for example on past landscapes and on plant responses to climate change. However, it meant that I was dealing only with plant parts that were long dead. My work was largely microscope based, often looking at plant material thousands of years old that had lost its original colour, shape and smell. Although fossilised plant material can be beautiful, especially fossil pollen (my favourites include daisy pollen, which, under a microscope, looks like a volcanic landscape, knotweed pollen grains, which are cratered like the moon, and the spiky asters and triangular myrtles), my day-to-day interaction with live plants amounted to little more than tending the sorry pots of basil on my kitchen windowsill or enjoying the trees that whizzed by as I cycled to work.

My professional relationship with plants expanded considerably when I became the founding director of Oxford University's Biodiversity Institute. The Institute – now part of the wider Oxford Biodiversity Network – used science to help provide the evidence for policy to protect the Earth's incredible biodiversity. My perspective became global: we were working to understand which ecological and evolutionary processes create the right conditions for resilience, persistence and the prevention of irreversible changes in ecosystems. And yet, my daily interaction with living plants did not increase significantly.

This all changed in 2013, when I went on secondment from Oxford to be Director of Science at the Royal Botanic Gardens, Kew in London. For those five years I was surrounded by living plants, from the lawns and borders of the public gardens outside my office window and the glasshouses containing palms from all over the world to the Japanese and Mediterranean gardens, and many more. I could travel the world in plants in a single lunch break. These daily interactions with plants changed the way I thought about them. I began to see plants in a totally different light from looking at them flat on the academic page or as large, abstract ecosystems. This was a parallel universe, all around me. And I was struck by how many visitors didn't just look at the plants or walk along beside them, but stopped to inhale their fragrances, bask in their shade, or reach out to touch leaves or stroke bark, ignoring those stern English signs telling them 'Do Not Touch' or 'Keep Off The Grass'. I ignored them too.

Over time, I ceased to seek out the Latin names for plants during my forays around the gardens at Kew or to try to determine which plant family they were in (not that I don't still enjoy this level of detail). Rather, I began to classify them in my own mind according to their stature, leaf shape, colour, scent, texture and even the sound the plant made in the breeze. I was no longer only seeing plants through a microscope lens, and with my attention focused on their complex role in an ecosystem, plants had become 'alive' to me, affecting all my senses.

Another thing I noticed during these lunchtime strolls was that I felt happier, calmer and more clear-headed – to the point that, even when extremely pressured for time, I still found the space to go walking in the gardens because it fostered a profound sense of well-being in me. And I couldn't help noticing that if I walked in the streets for the same length of time it did not have the same effect. It was something about the environment I was walking in.

I thought nothing more about these personal observations until I was asked to do some writing for an international project detailing the societal benefits we gain from plants. I was asked to find tangible examples of the health benefits derived from having plants in our everyday environments; for example, the role of city trees in removing particulate matter from the air, thus improving air quality.

As I trawled through the archives, I kept coming across mentions of a certain study which intrigued me. It was published in 1984 in the journal *Science*, and revealed the remarkable fact that patients recovering from gallbladder operations who could see trees from their hospital-bed windows recovered faster than those who looked onto brick walls.[1] They also had better post-operative mental well-being and required fewer doses of strong pain relief drugs. Amazingly, the authors concluded that just the *sight* of plants can have direct positive impacts on the patients' health. This study was different from all the others I had been reviewing because it suggested that it was not the plant itself affecting or altering the environment which triggered the positive health outcomes; instead, it was a more direct relationship between our experiencing plants through our senses (in this case seeing them) and the resulting health benefit.

My curiosity was awakened. The more I looked into this, the more published studies I came across showing that, along with sight, the effect of smelling, hearing and even touching certain plants can trigger measurable (and sometimes long-lasting) positive physical and mental health changes in us.

But haven't we known for a long time that interacting with plants is good for our well-being? Writers and philosophers through the ages have certainly thought so. For example, the Stoic school, established by the Greek philosopher Zeno of Citium in the fourth century BCE, proposed that in order to achieve a 'philosopher' state (in which a person becomes focused and can flourish), an individual needs to attune to nature. Gautama Buddha, around the sixth century BCE, made it a central proposition of Buddhism that meditation should be aligned to the rhythms of nature in order to gain enlightenment, with woods and forests being among the best places to meditate. Christian Gothic architecture built the shapes of trees and spreading branches into its soaring columns and vaults to draw the eyes of worshippers to heaven through the contemplation of natural images. And Romantic poets wrote about how 'the power/Of harmony' found in nature could provide 'tranquil restoration' from 'the din/Of towns and cities', as Wordsworth put it.

More recently Edward O. Wilson, the eminent Harvard ecology professor, suggested in his 1984 book *Biophilia* that our inherent affinity with nature is a deep evolutionary trait and a vital contributor to human health, productivity and well-being.[2] He proposed that we need to conserve and restore nature, not only for the material benefits that it can provide, but also for the positive influence certain aspects of it can have on our well-being.

But in recent decades strong voices have challenged the evolutionary hypothesis.[3] What, they ask, was the advantage to our early ancestors of being less stressed in green environments? While some green spaces may have represented opportunities for shelter and food, and hence less stress, it is hard to imagine how seeing a group of verdant green trees in a landscape quickly increased their chances of survival. Lack of clear scientific evidence to demonstrate the links between our sensing of plants and our health added strength to these voices of scepticism, with derogatory terms such as 'tree huggers' and 'voodoo science' sometimes assigned to those proposing such links.

The sceptics are now, however, gradually quietening. This is largely due to new innovations in scientific research that are starting to provide the elusive body of evidence for a direct link between positive health outcomes and the interaction of our various senses with plants. It certainly became quickly apparent through my research that a whole new branch of science is emerging that demonstrates an incredibly important medical link between sensing nature and our health.

This trend is illustrated through the story of *Shinrin-yoku* (森林浴), or 'forest bathing', in Japan. There are three Japanese characters which make up this word (森林浴). The first (森) is of a forest, represented by three trees. The second (林) is of a wood represented by two trees. The third represents bathing (浴), and depicts a house with flowing water on the left and a valley on the right. Shinrin-yoku literally means 'taking in the forest atmosphere through all our senses'. The word, and the actions it describes, sound like something that is steeped in a tradition going back hundreds, if not thousands, of years. In fact, the term was created in the 1980s as a marketing slogan to attract people to visit Japan's many beautiful forests. Despite the advertisers' confident puff, there was at this point little scientific data to support the suggestion that forest bathing actually had quantifiable health benefits.

It was only in the early 1990s that several notable teams of Japanese scientists set about scientifically testing this hypothesis.[4] This involved conducting a suite of medical and psychological tests on large numbers of participants, some of whom spent time walking or sitting in forests while others spent the equivalent amount of time doing the same things in an adjacent urban area. The results were startling. Walking for fifteen minutes in the forests compared to urban environments showed up to a 16 per cent reduction in the stress hormone cortisol in the participants' saliva, and a significant decrease in pulse rate and blood pressure. There was also a large increase in parasympathetic nerve activity (known to increase during times of relaxation) for those participants who walked or sat in the forests compared to urban areas. In addition, the participants reported feeling psychologically calmed, and noted an improvement in their overall mood when in the forests. Shinrin-yoku, thanks to new scientific evidence, was validated as a real phenomenon.

Since these early experiments, there has been a mushrooming of studies finding similar scientific evidence for important medical benefits to be gained from forest bathing.[5] And although these experiments have been predominantly carried out in Japan and China, benefits associated with forest bathing have also been demonstrated in other parts of Asia, Europe and the US, including evidence for improvements in the functioning of the immune system, the cardiovascular system and the respiratory system, as well as positive impacts on depression, anxiety and stress.

But do we need to be in forests to gain these effects, or can the same occur in city parks, walking in tree-planted urban streets or pottering in our back gardens? Thankfully, we are finally able to gather sufficient large-scale information to answer this question, and others, through the combined use of biobanks and satellite imagery.

Outside of the medical field, the term biobank is poorly known. Yet these 'banks' probably represent some of the most important collections of data to emerge in the past few decades for understanding trends and patterns in human health.

Population biobanks are, as their name suggests, collated samples of biological material (blood, DNA and so on) and records of individuals from across a population, not just those who are targeted because they have a particular disease. Individuals are invited to join these population biobanks and to have their personal data, medical records and tissue samples recorded. There are also some data repositories that simply collate publicly available details (e.g. mortality and cause of death). As a result, these banks represent a snapshot of the population, spanning different ages, gender, socio-economic groups and locations. Many countries now have or are developing these banks of population health data, and their potential to improve our understanding of the links between human health and the environment is huge.

Population biobanks have developed alongside another incredibly important data source: environmental sensors on satellites. These sensors are able to capture continental-scale environmental pictures at very fine scale (where images (pixels) are captured globally at a resolution of every thirty metres (100 feet) or less). One particularly useful satellite measurement in terms of understanding the relationship between health and natural features is the 'Normalised Difference Vegetation Index', or NDVI, which measures the health, or 'vigour', and greenness of the vegetation in any given place. NDVI is calculated by looking at the difference in the amount of visible 'red light' (healthy plants) versus 'near infrared light' (dying plants) that is reflected from vegetation.

NDVI measurements have revealed some of the most intriguing correlations between the environment and human health. For example, the greener the environment in which your house is situated, the less depressed you are.[6] A landmark study which used NDVI and the UK biobank revealed the significant protective effect of green environments against depression, and showed that, even after taking into account factors such as age, socio-economic status and cultural differences, the incidence of diagnosis and treatment of mental health disorders is less the greener the environment people live in. The effects were more pronounced among women, especially those under sixty years of age and in areas with low socio-economic status or higher urbanicity. Similar study findings, albeit with smaller sample sizes, have also been reported in cities in the US, Spain, France and South Africa.

Another study using large-scale population health data alongside satellite data found a link between the death of millions of city street trees and more than 21,000 additional human deaths due to respiratory illness and cardiovascular incidents.[7] The study asked an interesting question: if you remove the trees from city streets – thereby eliminating their beautiful green canopies – does it have a negative impact on human health? It examined what happened to cardiovascular and lower-respiratory-tract illness as a fast-moving infestation of the emerald ash borer killed street trees in US cities within two years of infestation. This infestation moved across the US in the 2000s in a wave-like pattern from east to west, killing over 100 million ash trees. By comparing the timing and location of the death of these trees with geolocated public health mortality records at the county level, these two big datasets revealed that an additional 6,113 human deaths related to respiratory illness and an additional 15,080 cardiovascular-related deaths occurred across the country as successive counties became infested. The magnitude of this effect became greater as the infestation progressed and was particularly pronounced in counties with above-average median household income.

Taken together, these two exciting advancements in data collection are providing a treasure-trove of specific information that can be used to scientifically compare an individual's medical records, and any diseases they might have, with the environment in which they live. These study results illustrate the power of these datasets to analyse data in ways that were not possible before. Why is this information important? Because it has profound implications for us as individuals, and for policy makers who are grappling with the startling statistics of public health epidemics, cardiovascular disease, respiratory illness, increased anxiety, depression and suicide. In the UK alone, 7.6 million people are currently living with cardiovascular disease: globally, it is the leading cause of death. And currently around 15 per cent of the UK population are taking antidepressants. The information now available to us provides another weapon in our armoury in the fight to combat these modern-day plagues and health crises. The recommended solutions are simple, economical and easy for anyone to do. The prescription is nature.

However, as important as the large data studies have been in establishing the relationship between plants and human health, they haven't been able to explain what is actually happening to our bodies when our senses interact with plants. All they can do is illustrate an association, not the causal link. This is where the real forensic work began for me, and this is an important focus of this book. It is a search to understand *how* we are physically and mentally affected when our senses of sight, sound, smell and touch interact with nature.

Delving into all the fascinating work being done in this area over the last decade or so started a very different academic endeavour for me. I wanted to know what actually happens in our brains, to our hormones and to our immune, respiratory and cardiovascular systems when we interact with plants – and which senses are triggered to bring about these reactions. I also wanted to know the best way to interact with plants both outdoors and indoors to gain the maximum physiological and psychological health benefits.

This academic journey has taken me far and wide. The people undertaking this research include not only plant scientists and biologists, but also medical practitioners, psychiatrists, city planners and government health authorities. They come from many countries, but they all share a common aim: they want to use science to discover the precise mechanisms by which our interacting with nature can bring about positive health outcomes, and then to use this knowledge to alter how we build nature into our daily lives and into public policy.

This book will take you with me on my quest to understand which aspects of seeing, smelling, touching or hearing nature bring about positive health outcomes – and where there are knowledge gaps that need to be filled. It will also take you on my personal journey – how I came to better appreciate our natural environment as being critical to my health and well-being. This journey has also renewed my passion to care for our planet's many diverse green environments, and to focus public policy on promoting and protecting more green spaces, especially among urban landscapes where the need is greatest. I hope that by the end of this book, we will all feel like specialists in this area of science and use the knowledge to influence our daily decisions about how best to immerse ourselves in the beauty and calming effect of plants and green spaces.

As a final note, one positive thing to emerge from the Covid pandemic was the renewed desire to spend time in nature. Visitor numbers to public gardens, parks and woodlands soared across the world. There was a huge surge in gardening and in sales of houseplants. It would appear that when things got grim and depressing, our species re-discovered an inherent need to be close to and surrounded by nature. This book will reveal why that is. I hope that, when you put it down, you will see tree-hugging in a whole new light.

1

Green Horizons: Why the View Matters

We've all seen the movie: the teenage protagonist feels out of place at school and stares out of the classroom window, their attention distracted by waving trees and squabbling ducks in the nearby park, until dragged back to the breeze-block reality of the interior of the classroom by a sarcastic remark from the teacher.

I suspect the urge to stare out of the window is in all of us, particularly if we are looking at a green vista. So, what's going on here? Why are we distracted by views of nature from a classroom or workspace? Is this distraction instinct trying to tell us something? And does the character of the landscape make a difference to its power to take us out of the here and now, if only for a moment?

Let's give the question a brief historical twist. In the Renaissance and early modern periods, garden design in England, and across Europe, was based on formality and order, on straight lines and practical things like kitchen gardens, orchards and fish ponds. In the early eighteenth century the emerging discipline of English landscape design changed all that. First, William Kent 'leapt the fence and saw that all nature was a garden'. Then came Lancelot 'Capability' Brown. Brown blurred the boundaries between art and nature. He believed that we derive greater pleasure from looking at carefully crafted but naturalistic scenes of rolling parkland dotted with individual trees, winding rivers crossed by elegant stone bridges, and a distant vista of a green horizon. His work was enormously popular, his services hugely in demand: no fewer than 270 gardens are attributed to him.

Today, we still flock to spend time in the gardens and parks he created. I certainly do. I often walk with my family and our dogs in the parks at Blenheim and Stowe, not far from where I live. Last summer we spent a wonderful afternoon at Chatsworth in Derbyshire. All three parks were designed and built by Brown and display the same characteristics of green views across open landscapes with a scattering of trees interspersed by the occasional glimpse of a building or a lake.

As the Duke of Devonshire, who owns and lives at Chatsworth, said in an interview in 2016, 'I don't think visitors care whether the landscape is real or not real – it just is. When you think of all the unlovely parts of life, to come to a place like this for a bit of quiet contemplation and mental refurbishment means a great deal to people.'[1]

But does this 'mental refurbishment' do us good in a measurable, quantifiable way? And are some views better than others and, if so, why? This is where my quest for answers begins.

In 2016 a team of researchers from the University of Illinois set out to ask whether the type of view seen from the classroom window had any effect on the cognitive function and attainment levels of students (although history doesn't record if they set out on this path because they were fed up with their own students staring out of the window).[2]

Ninety-four students from five high schools were randomly assigned to one of three classrooms. These rooms were of almost identical size, shape, lighting and furniture, but each had a different view: one looked out onto green space with trees, the second looked onto a blank wall, and the third had no windows at all. The children sat in chairs facing the window or wall and completed activities specifically designed to assess their attention functioning, including a proof-reading test, a speech test and a subtraction test. While doing so their levels of stress were recorded using measurements of body temperature, heart-rate variability and skin conductance, which can be used as a measure of stress because when we feel anxious sweat gland activity increases, which in turn increases skin conductance.

Intriguingly, even though all the children started with the same baseline levels of attention functioning and physiological stress, there were clear differences by the end of the task. Those who had a view of nature and green space from the window showed much better results in the tests than those in the rooms with no window or who looked out onto a blank wall. They also recovered much faster from elevated stress levels caused by the test.

Even after considering possible confounding variables such as cultural and socio-economic factors, the findings remained statistically strong and important; children who could see green views from their window had better-directed attention and recovered faster from raised levels of stress. Importantly, it also showed that the children did not need to be entirely immersed in nature to obtain these benefits – they just needed to see nature from their classroom window.

And this response is not just seen in children. In another study, university students showed significantly lower errors in a test and reported feeling more mentally restored after just a forty-second view of a flowering green roof from the window. In effect their attention and recovery from mental fatigue were greatly improved, compared to when they viewed a bare concrete roof for the same length of time.[3] Even a visual micro-break, for a very short interval of time, appears to be effective.

So, what is triggering these sorts of changes in us when we view natural landscapes?

Start with the basics of the biology of vision, learnt (in my case at least) some years ago in the kind of classroom where we began this chapter. When we look at something, light passes through the cornea (the clear bit in the front of the eye), then through the pupil (the hole in the coloured iris) and hits the lens. The lens then focuses the light onto the retina at the back of the eye. The retina is a layer of photoreceptive cells, and these turn the light into electrical signals which travel via the optic nerve to the brain, where the image is translated into what we see. Muscles in the eye also change the shape of the lens, allowing us to focus on things that are either near or far away.

What I didn't know until beginning to research this topic is that when we look at something, our eyes follow a distinctive pattern of scanning and then fixation. Eye-tracking technology (a combination of infrared and visual cameras which follow the movements of our eyes when exposed to external stimuli – i.e. when looking at something) has revealed that our eyes follow a coarse-to-fine strategy when we look at pictures, architecture and nature. First, they scan the overall picture, and then they focus in, scrutinising the finer detail of the scene and fixing on certain points. During each fixation our eyes select the most relevant information, and then integrate its features (shape, colour, orientation) to form a perception of the object. Our brain translates this visual information into images. This is when a number of physiological and psychological responses are triggered, depending on the shape, arrangement and colour of the images viewed. For example, seeing a large ferocious dog hurtling towards us might trigger both an elevated stress response, and a muscle response making our legs run (at least, we hope it does). A calm verdant scene might trigger the opposite response.

Understanding the causes of elevated stress in our bodies, and, on the flip side, what makes us less stressed, is an emerging branch of medicine. This is because high stress makes us more susceptible to a whole plethora of sicknesses. These include heart attacks, strokes, cancers, diseases associated with impaired inflammatory/immune responses, fatigue and depression.[4]

Stress is manifest in our bodies through three main and often interconnected pathways. First, when we are stressed, changes occur in our nervous system (brain, spinal cord and peripheral nerves), triggering involuntary changes to our breathing rate, heart-rate variability and width (narrowing) of blood vessels. Second, stress can trigger our endocrine system to release hormones such as cortisol and adrenaline from our glands to mobilise energy sources and increase our heart rate and blood pressure. Third, when we are stressed, this can affect our psychological state, with anxiety, depression and low moods being the most common symptoms.

Given all of these adverse effects, understanding how to reduce and manage stress is an important branch of medicine. Common medications to manage symptoms of stress include tranquillisers, beta-blockers, antidepressants and selective serotonin reuptake inhibitors (SSRIs), among others. But increasingly, health-care practitioners are starting to explore other approaches and treatments, to both prevent stress occurring in the first place, and also reduce elevated levels. And this is where taking time to view natural scenes on the horizon is revealing some fascinating findings.

The first finding is that when we look at a natural landscape scene compared to an urban one, even on a computer, we become calmer. For example, in a study by a team of scientists from the Centre for Environment, Health and Field Sciences in Chiba University, they asked female students to look at photos of a forest and of high-rise office blocks for just ninety seconds each. Clear results emerged:[5] when viewing the natural scene photo, physiological calming was evidenced in their brain activity, and psychological relaxation was recorded in students' responses to the questionnaires, with these indicating increased perceptions of feeling 'comfortable', 'relaxed' and 'natural'. It would appear that viewing natural scenes can trigger pathways in our bodies that make us calmer and less anxious. However, this study, and a number of others showing similar findings, involved healthy individuals who were sitting in a quiet room looking at images on a computer screen – hardly the sort of environment that most often results in us being stressed. So do we get the same reactions in more 'real life' stressed situations such as in a highly pressurised workplace?

And this is where a second interesting finding is emerging. A large number of studies are now showing that when we are stressed, we recover much quicker if we look at natural rather than urban scenes. A nice example of this is the findings of an experiment where office staff were asked to sit at a desk for ten minutes and view either a set of slides showing nature scenes typical of those you might see from an office window (trees, open grasslands), or of built environments (office blocks, streets with cars and so on).[6] They then underwent a five-minute activity to elevate levels of mental and physical stress. This involved studying a series of numbers on a screen and having ten seconds to write them down in the correct order. The participants were told that a buzzer would sound each time an incorrect answer was given. In fact, and somewhat unfairly I think, the buzzer was sounded twice during the test irrespective of whether they got the answer right or not. This would definitely stress me out. The participants had continuous measurements taken of their breathing (frequency and depth), blood pressure and heart-rate variability to measure their physiological indicators of stress. They also filled in two psychological questionnaires, one before and one after the stress test.

The results were intriguing. As expected, all participants showed elevated levels of stress during the test. But those who had viewed scenes of nature beforehand showed significantly faster recovery rates from the stressful incident compared to those who viewed the urban scenes. They also showed less psychological stress.

The take-home message from this, of course, is that we should all look at natural scenes either out of the window or as photos on our computer screen if we are about to encounter a stressful situation at work. But how does it work? Why do we get faster recovery rates when looking at natural scenes?

To explain this, a leading environmental psychologist called Roger Ulrich and colleagues proposed the so-called Stress Reduction Theory (SRT) in the early 1990s.[7] They argued that we have two biologically predetermined responses to viewing nature. First, we have a preference for, and instinctively pay attention to, natural scenes. Second, when we do so, it leads to a more 'positively toned emotional state'. Together, these will trigger automatic physiological responses in our bodies when we view natural scenes, which cause us to recover faster from stress. In contrast, they argued that the same does not happen when we view urban environments – instead these can hamper recuperation, especially after stressful events. Since it was first proposed, many studies have tested this theory and shown it to be broadly correct – when we view natural environments, even from indoors, physiological indicators of stress in our bodies show faster rates of recovery.[8]

Fascinating stuff – never before has looking out of the window onto the garden seemed such an attractive pastime. However, another equally important thing that appears to happen when we look at natural scenes is that it improves our mental ability associated with certain tasks – or so-called cognitive functioning.

Cognitive functioning refers to the processes of learning, thinking, reasoning, remembering, problem-solving, decision-making and attention. While some of our cognitive functions decline as we get older, many change very little across our life span: and some, such as vocabulary, may even improve in later life. Cognitive functioning and performance also vary greatly between individuals, whether they are children, adolescents or adults. Of most relevance here, however, is the fact that some aspects can be improved at whatever age – and this is where studies showing how our cognitive function changes when we see natural views on the horizon are important. Fascinatingly, it would appear from a large body of emerging research that if we view natural compared to urban scenes when taking breaks, we see significant improvements in our working memory, attention control and cognitive flexibility (our ability to switch between thinking about two different concepts or to think about multiple concepts simultaneously).[9] Importantly, this is apparent in all age groups – it is never too late to start staring out of the window! – but some of the most interesting studies are those involving school-aged children. I will mention just one here to give a flavour of the data that is emerging.

This study was carried out in 2015 by a team of scientists led by Payam Dadvand, a research professor at the Barcelona Institute for Global Health in Spain.[10] Dadvand examined whether there was a difference in the cognitive development of primary school children who saw natural scenes on a daily basis. The quantity of natural green space that the children encountered in their everyday lives was measured using satellite imagery. Three areas were mapped; a 250-metre (275 yards) buffer around each child's home; a fifty-metre (fifty-five yards) buffer around the children's school buildings; and the amount of natural green space the child would encounter in their commuting route to school. The experiment was carried out over an entire school year, between 2012 and 2013, and involved 2,593 primary school children with an average age of 8.5 years old from thirty-six schools. While the neighbourhoods of the schools were all similar in terms of socio-economic factors, additional data on maternal education, parental employment, marital status and ethnicity were collected to understand if these variables would influence the outcome. The cognitive development of the children was measured over a year, with tests undertaken every three months to assess working memory and attention.

Remarkably, their findings showed that, regardless of socio-economic factors or family background, the greater the amount of natural green space that the children encountered in their everyday lives, the better their monthly progress in working memory and attentiveness. Possibly even more important was the finding that the strongest measure for improved cognitive performance was the amount of green space surrounding the children's school buildings, not on their commuting route. The authors suggested that this was most likely to be reflecting the fact that, since children spend most of their day at school inside, seeing natural scenes through the windows will therefore have most influence on improving their cognitive

Superior working memory

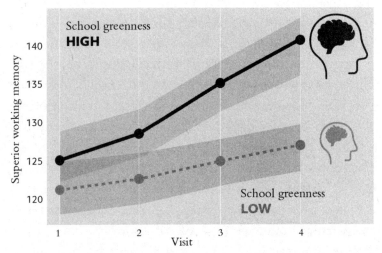

Source: P. Dadvand et al.

performance.[11] This has important policy implications for the design and location of schools.

But why do we see these clear improvements in cognitive function when we look at natural scenes? What is the process responsible? Explanations have been suggested in a theory from the field of the psychology of natural scenes, called Attention Restoration Theory. This was proposed by two professors of psychology at the University of Michigan, Stephen and Rachel Kaplan, in a set of seminal papers published in 1989 and 1995.[12] They hypothesised that views of nature improve our cognitive functioning because of the restorative effect that they have on our directed attention.

In our everyday lives our brains rely heavily on cognitive resources that direct attention towards a task that requires focus, while simultaneously ignoring background distractions such as people chatting and computers beeping to remind us that we have new emails. In psychology this cognitive resource is known as directed attention. However, our capacity to direct attention in this way cannot be sustained indefinitely, which is why our ability to concentrate tends to wax and wane during the day. Prolonged directed attention also leads to a state of mental fatigue, which is something we need to avoid as it is associated with, for example, poorer decision making, more errors and lower levels of self-control.

The Attention Restoration Theory proposes that seeing scenes of nature restores our directed attention, because viewing natural scenes draws instead upon our involuntary attention. This is when our mind is diverted (distracted) towards some other activity, for example something glimpsed in our peripheral field of vision, rather than being consciously and deliberately selected or focused on by us. But why do natural scenes draw on our involuntary attention more? The Kaplans propose that this is because, counter-intuitively, they contain far *fewer* stimuli that require our notice. So, when we are looking at natural scenes, our directed attention is given a 'mini-break', allowing it to recover and replenish. When we then return to tasks that require focus, we show better cognitive performance because our directed attention has recovered.[13]

To summarise: there appears to be a strong body of evidence showing that looking at natural scenes triggers psychological and physiological responses that bring about calming, faster recovery from stress and improvement in our working memory and attention. Explanations have been proposed in two foundational hypotheses on the psychology of natural scenes, as mentioned above: Stress Reduction Theory and Attention Restoration Theory.

The studies I have mentioned up to this point have been binary in terms of landscape types: natural or urban. But of course, nature comes in infinite variety: tropical rainforests dense with vegetation, flat grasslands, scattered trees on a savanna landscape. Every day we look at the different shapes of tree canopies, probably without a second thought, yet they create a distinctive set of shapes in any landscape. Just looking out of my window as I type this, I can see a copper beech with its globular-shaped canopy, a tall, thin, almost spindly shaped silver birch, and two conical-shaped conifers in my neighbour's garden. Are some of these shapes and/or the landscapes they are situated upon (such as those designed by Capability Brown) better to look at for the health benefits that they provide?

When most of us think of a plant, we probably picture an upright structure (stem) with branches and leaves at the end of them. Rarely will we think of algae, moss or hornwort – even though these are also plants. The plants we are thinking of are instead vascular plants. These have a system of specialised cells which contain the biological equivalent of a strengthening agent called lignin. Evidence for its presence in plants first appears in the fossil record around 400 million years ago.[14] And it was this innovation, along with a few others, that resulted in a development from toe-brushing floppy plant specimens, which first inhabited Earth around 480 million years ago, to upright herbs, shrubs and tree-like structures, some up to ten metres in height. I find it incredible that this all happened within a mere 100 million years which, even though on human timescales it sounds like a long time, is in fact amazingly short in geological timescales.

These early landscapes contained many tree types that have long gone extinct. But if we took a walk in them, it would probably not be the branches, leaves or stems of these early trees that would tell us that we had made a mistake in our time-travel machine and got out in the wrong geological time period, but their strange combinations. In fact, some of these tree types remind me of a childhood board game called 'Guess Who?' where, by asking questions and selecting cards showing different facial features such as eyes, noses, hair and so on, you can work out the character. If you get it wrong, you create a very odd-looking person. To me, these early tree forms look as if someone has been playing the plant equivalent and made many mistakes; six-metre-high (twenty-foot-high) horsetail trees, similar to our tiny horsetail plants we see today (*Equisetum*) but in tree form and with leaf branches in whorled structures up their stem; ten-metre (thirty-three-foot) lycopod trees (*Lepidodendron*) with distinctive diamond-shaped patterned bark but a flourish of fern-like fronds poking out of the top of their long trunks; and eight-metre (twenty-six-foot) *Cordaites* trees, with a branching structure similar in outline to many present-day deciduous trees, but long thin leaves similar in shape and size to those we see in the modern iris plant family (*Iridaceae*).

Most of these early trees reproduced using spores, a mode of reproduction akin to present-day ferns, whose spores you can see on the underside of the fronds, and which are then distributed by the wind. Tree ferns were also in these early landscapes but often around three times taller than what we are used to now. Some trees, however, are very similar to those we see today including conifers, araucaria, ginkgoes and cycads. In fact, there are many tree species in our landscapes today for which we have evidence from the fossil record to indicate that nearly identical forms existed over 350 million years ago. These so-called 'living fossils' in the plant kingdom are far more common than in the animal kingdom, where predecessors existed in very different forms (for example dinosaurs).

The broad variety of vegetation types that we see on our global landscapes now was established by around seventy million years ago. Despite various subsequent changes and extinctions, this means that the plants we see around us are very similar in size and shape to those our first ancestors (species *Homo sapiens*) would have encountered on the African landscapes in which they evolved around 300,000 years ago. They would also have seen similar outlines of tree shapes resulting from the branching pattern, the height at which the branching occurs, length and straightness of the branches and their angle of divergence. It is these characteristics that influence the overall shape and look of trees, resulting in tree canopy shapes which can be broadly defined as conical, spreading, columnar, rounded, oval or fan-shaped. What is also interesting is that these contrasting tree shapes are unevenly distributed across the globe, in distinctive assemblages of vegetation resulting from differences in climate and other factors such as frequency of fire events

Common characteristic tree shapes

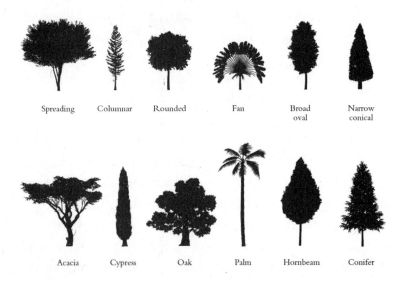

Spreading	Columnar	Rounded	Fan	Broad oval	Narrow conical

Acacia	Cypress	Oak	Palm	Hornbeam	Conifer

and amounts of herbivory. Their density on landscapes also varies greatly from a few scattered trees in savannas, to more open broad-leaved woodlands containing a mosaic of trees and other shrubs, to large dense coniferous forests.

The location of these different vegetation assemblages are determined primarily by climate, so in regions that have similar climates, similar occurrences of vegetation are found – despite sometimes being in totally different parts of the world; for example, the 'Mediterranean biome' can be found in California, south-western Australia, south-eastern Chile and South Africa as well as in southern Europe.

These distinctive biome assemblages are not a recent landscape feature – they can be identified in fossil records as far back as 300 million years ago, altering and changing in terms of geographical location, extent and plant composition in response to major climatic events such as tectonic plate movements, meteorite impacts and volcanic eruptions. The arrangement of biomes we currently find across the globe became established around ten million years ago. This means that the natural landscapes that we see today, from dense coniferous forests to open grasslands, are similar to those our earliest ancestors would have lived in. In particular, fossil evidence shows the early landscapes of our ancestors were open savanna landscapes, punctuated with scattered trees, such as *Acacia*, which has a characteristic short trunk and a dense spreading canopy.

Some have even gone as far to suggest that we have we have a preference for the tree shapes and styles of early savanna landscapes 'in our genes'.[15] Why? Because, they argue, the selective pressures imposed on early humans in Africa, specifically in the savanna environments, were so important for their survival that we still have an innate preference for them. And strange though it may first seem, a number of studies appear to show that we do have some quite strongly aligned preferences, regardless of our age or background, for certain tree and landscape shapes. For example, when 277 students from University of California, Davis were asked to view six different computer-generated silhouettes of tree shapes (spreading, columnar, globe-shaped, fan shaped, broad oval and narrow conical) and select their preference for height and width, there emerged remarkable consistency in their selection.[16] Short-trunked trees with a large width to height ratio (think acacia and oak trees) were the most liked, with pointy-shaped conifer trees showing the lowest preference ratings. Similar findings have been found in participants from many different cultures, ages and socio-economic backgrounds.[17] It would therefore appear that many of us prefer looking at deciduous trees with a short trunk height and a wide spreading canopy.

Of course, when we look at a landscape we are not just looking at the shape of an individual tree, but at the setting in which it sits. Most natural views are made up of a combination of open space and different kinds of trees and other plants. Personally, I'm a big fan of open vistas with a few scattered trees such as oak. But is this because I grew up in the rolling hills of the temperate south-east of England where this sort of landscape occurs naturally, or because I have a deep-seated innate preference for seeing savanna-like horizons resulting from ancient genes that I have inherited from my African ancestors? I had always assumed the former, but a number of studies have left me wondering.

For example, when research scientists John Balling and John Falk from Oregon State University asked 545 participants to view and score a series of different landscape types from over the world based on how much they would like to live in and visit them, remarkably consistent responses emerged.[18] Even though the participants ranged in age from third to ninth grade school children (eight to sixteen years) through to university students, working professionals and retired senior citizens, they all rated savanna landscapes highly. In fact, they were rated as strongly as the photos which depicted landscapes of more familiar surroundings in Washington DC and Maryland. Probably the most interesting finding was that children under the age of twelve showed the strongest preference for these savanna landscapes, when few of them had ever visited or even seen pictures of these types of landscape before.

However, the proposal that we have a deep-seated evolutionary preference harking back to the savanna-like landscapes in which we evolved is not without its critics. There has been fair criticism that the participants in the studies tend to have come from US-European and urban-dwelling populations. These individuals have typically lived in cities where the landscapes that surround them could be said to be savanna-like in their structure (i.e. a few trees scattered on a predominantly open landscape, even if the climate conditions are not savanna-like), so their preference might well be based on current personal experience, not an evolutionary legacy.[19] To test this suggestion Balling and Falk therefore did a follow-on study in 2010 using participants who had lived their whole life in the rainforest belt of Nigeria.[20] These included children based in a co-educational school surrounded by remnant patches of tropical rainforest, teenagers from a school located in a small fishing village on one of the islands in the Niger delta, and young adults who studied at a technical college, but whose homes were surrounded by tropical rainforest.

Seventy-three per cent of the participants had never travelled outside the rainforest biome of West Africa. Similar to the previous experiment, they were asked to score photos of different landscapes according to preference and how much they would like to live in the environment. Intriguingly, responses from the vast majority of the participants still indicated a strong preference for the pictures of savanna landscapes. So, even though their homes were surrounded by tropical rainforest, and most had never visited the savanna, they still preferred these open landscapes.

This study hints that we may indeed have an innate preference for savanna-like settings, possibly representing a vestigial trait of our evolution in the savannas of East Africa. However, a serious note of caution must be added here. Several studies using similar approaches carried out since 2010 have reported contrasting findings, suggesting that this topic requires more research and much larger sample sizes before any firm conclusions on the 'out-of-Africa' preference hypothesis can be safely drawn.[21]

But we also need to be careful more broadly not to get too bogged down in theories of evolutionary psychology, because in some ways this is missing the point. What we really need to know is: does an open view with scattered trees on the horizon result in better physiological and psychological outcomes when we view it compared to other landscape scenes?

It was while looking for answers to this question that I discovered some of the most interesting research on this topic to date.

At the beginning of the chapter, I mentioned when describing the basics of eye biology that, when we look at something, our eyes follow a distinctive pattern of scanning and then fixation. What I didn't go on to mention is the discovery that our eyes also appear to seek out patterns with a mid-level of *fractal* complexity.[22] Why is this significant? Because evidence suggests that when we view silhouette outlines of natural scenes with this fractal dimension, it triggers greater levels of calming and attention restoration than when we look at the outline shape of other landscape types.

To unpack this and its significance, we first need a bit of explanation about fractals. The word comes from the Latin *fractus*, which means broken or fractured. It is used specifically to describe shapes that have patterns that repeat when viewed at increasingly fine magnifications. For example, when you look at a coastline on a large-scale map (1:10,000), you see the broad outline of bays interspersed by headlands. If you focus down to view the coastline pattern on a medium-scale map (1:5,000), you see smaller bays and inlets within the larger pattern, and zooming in further to a fine resolution map (1:2,000), there will also be smaller inlets, and so on down to the level of rock pools and patterns in the sand on a beach. These bays and headlands are broadly the same shape but each time you zoom in they are smaller and fit within the larger shape.

The number of times you have a repeating pattern within a larger pattern, or in other words its visual complexity, is called its fractal dimension. This is a ratio providing a statistical measure of the visual complexity (D-value) that has values ranging between 1 and 2. The greater the number of repeating patterns, the closer the D-value to 2. For example, a straight line has a D-value of 1, whereas a line with a multiple repeating pattern of wobbles in it recurring at finer and finer scales will be closer to 2.[23] Fractals are found in many features of everyday life: in art, architecture and importantly in natural scenes.[24] Trees, for example, are inherently fractal in their shape, with larger

Fractal dimension of three contrasting horizons

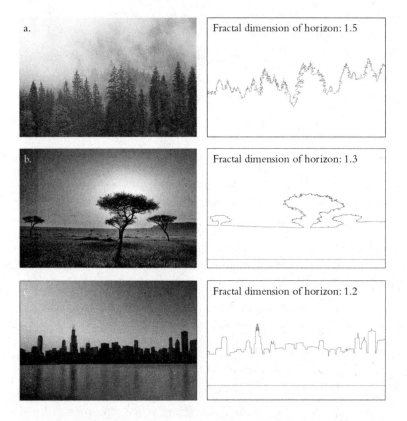

a.

Fractal dimension of horizon: 1.5

b.

Fractal dimension of horizon: 1.3

Fractal dimension of horizon: 1.2

branching patterns seen repeated in smaller branches, twigs and even right down to small twiglets.

But the real significance of fractals for our purposes is when we look at the outline of natural scenes on the horizon. Seminal work carried out in the early 2000s by Richard Taylor, a physicist from the University of Oregon, showed that when we are looking at pictures, our eyes are seeking out (in their fixation pattern) a fractal dimension of between 1.3 and 1.5. So that, despite looking at really complicated pictures, our eyes are still seeking this type of pattern with this mid-level of complexity. Even more extraordinarily, he then went on to demonstrate that regardless of whether it was a computer-generated image, a photo or a painting, we still have a strong preference for images that have this level of visual complexity.[25] For example, when 199 participants randomly sampled from the general public were asked to view fifty-two different landscape scenes, which were all normalised to black and white so that colour was not an influence, there was a strong preference for images that had a fractal outline silhouette of 1.3.[26] What I find even more interesting is the fact that landscapes with this fractal dimension tend to be open landscapes with a few scattered trees.

It appears that we prefer these shapes. But does this preference lead to any perceptible health benefits? What happens to us when we see silhouette horizons with fractal complexity between 1.3 and 1.5?

This final piece of the jigsaw was completed by some exemplary studies carried out by Caroline Hägerhäll and colleagues from the Swedish University of Agricultural Sciences in 2006.[27] In these, they devised an experiment where participants had their brain activity measured via an electroencephalogram (EEG) while viewing different computer-generated pictures (i.e. not natural scenes – just silhouette outlines) of different fractal complexities. The EEG is a non-invasive test which requires the participants to wear a skull cap (similar to a bathing cap) containing holes through which electrodes are placed at certain points, touching the scalp surface. These electrodes detect electrical activity that occurs when neuron cells in the brain transmit information to other nerve cells, muscle cells or gland cells via a process called synaptic transmission.

Importantly, this method can distinguish between various frequencies (wavelengths) of electric current in our brains, each one known to be enhanced when we are in different physiological states. Alpha frequencies (with wavelengths of between 7.5 and 13 Hz), for example, are enhanced when we close our eyes and bring ourselves into a relaxed state; delta waves (wavelengths below 3 Hz) in comparison are associated with when we are asleep and are therefore usually used to measure depth of sleep; the stronger the levels of delta activity, the deeper the sleep. Beta waves (wavelengths above 13 Hz) are commonly observed when we are in a wakened state with increased external focus and attention.

The significance of understanding these different brain wave types becomes apparent when the results from Hagerhall's experiments are examined. When subjects viewed the image with a fractal dimension of 1.3 their brain wave activity showed heightened alpha and beta frequencies and reduced delta frequencies, indicating that the participants became more relaxed, with increased focus and attention, and less sleepy. This was not replicated when viewing the other images. And this finding, that seeing natural scenes with a fractal dimension of 1.3 induces calming and increased focus and attention, has since been verified in other studies.[28]

These experiments have therefore managed to elegantly piece together the scientific building blocks to demonstrate why open landscapes with a few scattered trees provide greater calming and attention restoration. It is because they have an intermediate level of fractal complexity.

Other scientists have taken this idea one step further, by asking whether looking at natural scenes of mid-level fractal complexity also improves our cognitive performance, with findings to suggest that it does. When a group of volunteers were asked to view pictures of urban (low-fractal complexity) and natural (mid-fractal complexity) scenes, response times to questions were faster when viewing those of mid-complexity. But this is just one study.[29] More work is needed to understand this relationship in detail.

Of course, all such observations may also work the other way round. If one type of landscape induces positive reactions in us, then other landscapes may have the opposite effect. Personally I am not that keen on dense woodlands or streets with too many trees. They make me feel stressed. So, is there a threshold for how many trees there are on a landscape before it ceases to be a good thing for stress recovery?

Preliminary studies suggest that there probably is. Researchers at the University of Illinois, for example, who ran an experiment in which participants watched a selection of 3D videos showing different densities of trees and shrubs in the street, ranging between 2 per cent and 62 per cent in the field of vision, found marked differences in their rate of recovery from an interval of deliberately induced heightened level of stress.[30] Those that viewed streets with a tree density of 2–24 per cent showed faster recovery rates as the density of street trees increased. However, when the street tree density reached 24–34 per cent there was no further improvement in the stress recovery rates. And, once tree density reached more than 34 per cent of the image, there was a negative relationship, with the participants showing a slowing down in recovery rates as the views of trees became denser, to the point where there was no effect visible.

Oddly, though, this worked only with men. The experiment found no relationship between density of trees and recovery rates from stress for the women participants. The authors suggest this might be because the timescales and rate of physiological response to stress may be different, and that women may require longer exposure to nature to experience comparable levels of recovery to men. This certainly requires further research. In any case, I suspect that it is women more than men who find too high a density of trees stressful, even on city streets. I know I do. Urban planners should take note.

So, to return to our opening scene of a classroom of distracted students staring out of a window, from my brief foray into the science on this topic it would appear that taking a short micro-break to gaze at a varied natural landscape, or even look at pictures or photos of natural scenes, is a good thing to do. It triggers physiological and psychological pathways in our bodies that lead to reduced levels of anxiety, faster recovery rates from stressful events and improved cognitive functioning.

But it would also seem that we need to be selective in what we look at, since there is considerable variation in this response depending on the type of landscape. Ideally we should look at open natural vistas with a few scattered low-height trees with wide-based canopies. This was the insight captured by 'Capability' Brown 300 years ago, as if he and his many imitators somehow subconsciously understood that these sorts of scenes are more relaxing and better for our mental equilibrium. Their insights still hold true today.

Finally, we should listen to our internal voices (and folk tales) telling us to avoid viewing dense, dark forests – these will probably elevate rather than decrease our stress levels. Red Riding Hood's mother was on to something.

2

Why Green is Good for Us, and Not Just in What We Eat

Some years ago I went with my family on a camping holiday across upstate New York, New England and into Canada. This is a landscape that has long captured the American imagination. The nineteenth-century naturalist and writer Henry David Thoreau spent two years living alone in a cabin deep in the woods near Walden Pond in Concord, Massachusetts, and recorded his impressions in a series of evocative and influential books, still widely read today.

He takes special care to describe the colours of nature: 'A single gentle rain makes the grass many *shades* greener'; 'The lowest and inmost leaves next the bole are, as usual, of the most delicate yellow and green, like the complexion of young men brought up in the house.'[1]

Thoreau was particularly attracted to the riot of greens, browns, reds, whites, yellows, crimsons and oranges which spreads across this landscape in autumn. 'October is the month for painted leaves,' he wrote. 'Their rich glow now flashes round the world.' He observed the tints and shades of particular species: 'By the 25th of September, the Red Maples generally are beginning to be ripe. Some large ones have been conspicuously changing for a week, and some single trees are now very brilliant.' 'If you wish to count the Scarlet Oaks, do it now.' In the woods of Maine: 'The spruce and cedar on its shores, hung with gray lichens, looked at a distance like the ghosts of trees … The tops of mountains are among the unfinished parts of the globe.'

Strikingly, Thoreau did not just limit his observations to describing this wonderful profusion of colour and shade but was interested in the effect it had on him, the observer, the spectator: 'We can never have enough of nature. We must be refreshed by the sight of inexhaustible vigor … We need to witness our own limits transgressed, and some life pasturing freely where we never wander.'

I still cherish my memories of our campsite deep in the woods outside Woodstock, the waterfalls and inlets around the peaceful Finger Lakes, the dramatic wooded shoreline either side of Niagara Falls with the USA on one side and Canada on the other, and the gentler landscapes of Ontario. My memories are also in vivid colour: the American beech (*Fagus grandifolia*), whose pale grey bark and bright green leaves play magic tricks with the sunlight filtering through from above, the sugar maple (*Acer saccharum*) with its foliage like fire in the fall, the lime trees (American basswood, *Tilia americana*) with leaves as big as dinner plates, and the shagbark hickory (*Carya ovata*) whose peeling bark offers a nesting place for bats and whose nuts are harvested by birds, squirrels and chipmunks (some of whom appeared to enjoy using them for a spot of target practice aimed at the roof of our camper van in the middle of the night).

My family and I did not live in a cabin for two years. Our camper van and running water would hardly have passed muster with the hardier souls of former years. But

I would like to think that we absorbed some of that spirit and life-force described so beautifully by Thoreau, that we returned home 'refreshed by the sight of inexhaustible vigor'. I certainly felt that way myself.

Nor do we have to head stateside to enjoy the colours of nature. Look around you: even a modest suburban garden like my own displays a more or less infinite gradation of different shades of green, from the bright new grass after rain to the dusky leaves of the ageing apple tree, and the green and white leaves of the silver birch tree.

Now look at a single leaf on a houseplant: even here the palette of shade and tint is often varied, sometimes highlighted with white, red and yellow, as if someone has taken a set of colouring pencils and traced out the patterns and networks of veins and vessels.

We clearly have a deep-seated attraction to the different colour palettes of nature. But what I wanted to understand was whether different plant colours have any effect upon our well-being when we look at them. And this is where a study carried out in the early 2000s by two researchers, Andy Kaufman and Virginia Lohr, from the University of Hawaii really got me thinking. They asked the simple question: does it matter what colour trees you plant in a garden in terms of the well-being outcomes?[2] To address this, they recruited forty-two participants between the ages of eighteen and sixty and from twelve countries to represent a good spread of ages and cultural backgrounds. All were asked to view eighteen tree images in a random order. The tree shape was exactly the same each time, but digitally altered so that the canopy was various shades of green, red, orange and yellow. When viewing these images,

43

the effect of seeing the different colours on their stress levels was recorded by measuring their skin conductance.

Even though the methodology was simple, remarkably clear results emerged. Stress levels were significantly lower when the participants viewed the green canopies compared to the other colours. It would appear that some colours of nature might influence our response to it more than others.

This is fascinating. It set me wondering if we could bring these insights down to the local, personal level, and work out if there are ideal colours and shades to include in our own gardens and choice of houseplants.

Understanding how different plant colours might contribute to our sense of well-being first requires a brief foray into how and why we see different plant colours.

The 'how' part is relatively straightforward. We see different colours thanks to the millions of light-sensitive cells, some shaped like rods and some like cones, which cover the retina in the back of our eye. These process the light entering our eyes into nerve impulses, which then pass via the optic nerve to our brain. The rods transmit mostly black and white information to the brain and are concentrated mostly around the edge of the retina, which is why our peripheral vision is less sharp and colourful. The cones, by contrast, are concentrated in the middle of the retina, and they are responsible for transmitting the information on the range of colours and shades to the brain.

Why we see different colours is slightly more complicated, especially when looking at plants. This is because there are many factors responsible for the colours we see. Around half of the sunlight that reaches Earth is composed of wavelengths of light that are visible to us, and each section

of the visible spectrum accounts for a different colour –
red, orange, yellow, green, blue, indigo and violet. When
this visible light hits an object, these different wavelengths
are either absorbed or reflected back, and it is the light
that is reflected back that enters our eyes. So, what we see
is reflected light. And the parts of the wavelength (and
therefore colours) that are reflected back depend on the
properties of the object that is doing the reflecting. In
plants there are at least three properties that influence the
colour that we see: plant pigments themselves, the presence
of waxes and hairs, and microstructural features.[3]

Plant pigments are specific molecules found in plant
cells. They play a number of essential roles, ranging from
capturing energy from the sun for photosynthesis, to growth
and development. However, they also have another feature:
different plant pigments reflect back different wavelengths
of light. The colour of leaves and other parts of the plant are
therefore strongly influenced by the types of pigments that
they contain. Most leaves, for example, are green because
they contain lots of the pigment chlorophyll. Even though
the pigment itself is colourless, its properties are such that
it absorbs red and blue wavelengths and reflects back green,
and this is what we then see – green leaves. In contrast, if
leaves contain a lot of the plant pigment carotenoid, they
will appear red to us because these pigments absorb green
and blue wavelengths of light, and reflect back orange
and red.

Another feature responsible for the colour of foliage
is uneven surfaces on the leaves caused by micro-ridges,
furrows, hairs and waxy scales. When light waves hit these
uneven surfaces it causes differential refraction (bending)

and scattering.[4] As a consequence, even though the material itself might be transparent, it will appear coloured because some wavelengths of light have been refracted and scattered. In the animal world a classic example of this structural colour is the wings of the tropical blue morpho butterfly (*Morpho* sp.), whose vivid blue is not due to the presence of pigments but rather to micro-scales on the wing's surface. These scales refract and scatter blue light, which is then reflected back to us, making the wings look blue. An example of this phenomenon in the plant world is the white undersides of some leaves on trees such as white poplar (*Populus alba*). This is due to waxy scales and/or small hairs found on the undersides of these leaves which scatter and reflect the light back at many different angles and all wavelengths, resulting in the white colour we see.

Finally, different colours and tones in plants occur as a result of microstructural features *inside* the plant leaves. Plant cells which are convex in shape, sometimes stacked in piles of three or four inside the cells, can generate a very intense colour and even an iridescent sheen by reflecting back wavelengths of light at different angles at each layer between the stacked cells.[5] The eye-catching brilliance of the leaves of some species of begonia (*Begonia pavonina*), for example, is as a result of this process.

The science behind nature's role as artist is fascinating and complex. So are the biological and neurological processes by which we sense and interpret the colours around us. So what changes or mechanisms are triggered in our bodies when we see different colours in plant foliage?

When I first started looking for experiments that addressed this question, the majority of studies I came across did not look at plant colour specifically, but rather at our responses to single blocks of colour. But even these simple experiments yielded some tantalising evidence, suggesting that seeing green compared to other colours can trigger positive emotional states and creativity.

One such experiment was carried out in 2012 by researchers from the University of Munich.[6] In this, 202 participants aged between fifteen and forty-five years, including both males and females, were shown a piece of paper with a green, black, red or blue rectangle on it, for three seconds, and then asked to perform a series of tasks in two minutes. These included writing down as many suggested uses of a tin can as they could think of, and looking at a pre-generated geometric figure and drawing as many different objects made from this shape as they could in the allocated time: both of these are well-established methodologies to measure creativity. The results were coded by independent markers who scored the first test according to whether the suggestions were common, uncommon, unusual or clever – gaining a higher score for those that were unusual or clever (more creative). The second test was scored by the number of different objects generated in the allocated time, with a higher score for more. Results from this experiment were highly statistically significant; regardless of the age and sex of the participants, those individuals who viewed the green rectangle before undertaking the tasks were much more creative in both tests than those who viewed white, grey, red or blue.

Another intriguing study on colour by scientists at the University of Essex asked what happens when we see different colours while exercising, in this case in a gym.[7]

Participants undertook three five-minute peak-power performance cycling tests on fixed bikes. While doing so they watched video footage of a rural cycling course that simulated cycling through a natural leafy environment. The only difference each time they took the test was that the video they watched was coloured differently: an unedited version (with natural green vegetation), monochrome (grey and white), or one that had a red filter applied. Psychological (mood state and perceived exertion) and physiological (heart rate, oxygen uptake, respiration rate) measurements were taken during the three exercise periods.

A result that might help many of us while doing these (frankly quite dreadful) short intervals of intensive exercise is that those participants who viewed green vegetation in comparison to other colours had better moods and were less conscious of the perceived exertion of exercising. In comparison, feelings of anger were the highest after viewing the image with the red filter. However, no clear physiological differences were apparent in cardiorespiratory measures when viewing different colours so the benefits of seeing green, at least from this study, were only related to mental health outcomes. So, sadly, there are no obvious physical beneficial shortcuts when viewing green while at the gym, but there is definitely evidence for some improvement in mental well-being.

What these experiments therefore suggest is that the colour green makes us more relaxed and creative and gives us a more positive outlook. But how much of this is related to personal preference for the colour rather than an involuntary response? Do we feel calmer, more creative and in a better mood because we prefer the colour? Or are these changes triggered involuntarily, so that we prefer the colour because of the effect it has on us? This is a tricky but important question.

Our ability to address this question (and many others) is thanks to recent developments in brain-scanning techniques. One of the most important of these is called functional Magnetic Resonance Imagery (fMRI). This works because of a natural feature which came as a bit of a surprise to me: de-oxygenated blood is paramagnetic, meaning it acts like a magnet in the presence of a magnetic field.[8] Oxygen in our blood provides energy to different organs via an iron-containing protein molecule called haemoglobin (known as oxyhaemoglobin). When the oxygen is delivered to an organ, this molecule becomes de-oxygenated (deoxyhaemoglobin) and takes on paramagnetic properties. The fMRI scanner, which contains a powerful magnetic loop, acts like a large magnet, and can measure areas of the brain where neural activity has occurred because there is a surge of deoxyhaemoglobin. This technology has transformed our ability to understand neural activity in our brains in response to various prompts, not least visual cues including colour.

And it was this technology that was used in an interesting study in 2019 which asked if there are certain regions of the brain which have stronger activation when passively viewing a particular colour.[9] The researchers then asked a second question: does this activation increase when viewing those colours for which we have a personal liking? In effect, what they were trying to do was tease apart two questions: first, whether we have an involuntary response when viewing certain colours; and second, is this response linked to our personal preference for these colours?

To address these questions, the participants were scanned using fMRI while viewing twenty-four different colours in varying hues. They were not required to make judgements about their preferences among the different colours, but, rather, they were given a task which involved the use of the colour being investigated. For example, they were asked to judge whether a coloured square viewed on a screen was at one of four possible orientations.

Second, and after the scanning part of the experiment, the participants took a colour preference task. This involved them viewing all the colours seen previously and rating them on a preference scale from 'not liking at all' to 'liking very much'.

Clear results emerged. fMRI imaging of the brain showed that when viewing green and blue colours during the tasks involving different coloured squares and the like, there was significantly more activity in the part of the brain called the posterior midline cortex compared to when they viewed other colours. This is the area of the brain involved in preferences and value judgements, emotion and social behaviour, attention, learning and motivation, and suggests that seeing blue and green colours triggers more brain activity in these regions. Really fascinating stuff. But what about our preference for certain colours? Well, what I found even more interesting in this experiment was the finding that in the colour preference test, the colours that showed the highest brain activity were those the participants said they liked the most: the higher the spikes in neural activity in the brain, the more liked the colour in the preference test.

What this experiment elegantly demonstrates is that viewing green and blue colours seems to automatically trigger neural activity in areas of our brains associated with enhanced attentional and cognitive processes.[10] It also shows that there is a neural basis for our preference of these colours: the colours we like are those that trigger these reactions, not the other way around.

Of course in nature we are not just seeing single blocks of colour, but foliage of varying shades, often containing two or three colours on a single leaf. So, is there an 'ideal' mix of colours to look at for our mental and physical well-being?

Two-coloured or even multi-coloured plant leaves are especially common in houseplants, which indeed are often selected and marketed because of this feature. As I write this, I can see plants on my desk with white and green vertically striped leaves (a spider plant, *Chlorophytum comosum*), green leaves with red veins in a net-like pattern (nerve plant, *Fittonia verschaffeltii*), a poinsettia (*Euphorbia pulcherrima*) with leaves with red and green patterning and white-green ivy leaves (*Hedera helix*). I have these on my desk because I find them fascinating to look at. They illustrate an intricacy and beauty of colour combinations in nature that is akin to seeing the patterns on leopard or zebra skins but are far more practical (and safe) to have sitting on your desk. Although, come to think of it, I do like the idea of a zebra sitting by my side as I type this. But I digress. Can we say that any one of these colour combinations is better to look at for its health benefits?

In addition to the processes responsible for plant colouring mentioned above, two-toned colouring in leaves results from one further biological tweak: genetic mutations. These can alter the colour of the pigment in cells in the plant's meristem tissue. The meristem tissue is found in the parts of the plant responsible for growth, usually in the tips of the roots and shoots, the stem and growing leaves. It contains layers of actively dividing cells, and this is how these parts of the plant grow. The cells in the meristem tissue are switched on (or off) by a growth hormone called auxin and this triggers them to start dividing at certain times in response, for example, to increasing levels of light associated with the coming of spring.

Any genetic mutations that occur in the first layer of these meristem cells, therefore, will be carried on into the next cell through cell division, and so on. And this is particularly well seen in plant colouration, because any pigment alternation, which changes the colour of meristem tissue from green to white, for example, will be carried on throughout the developing leaf. Therefore, as the leaf grows, these white sections of tissue in the leaf will divide and be apparent as a white pattern on a green leaf. The same process is also true for many other patterned colours on green leaves; they represent a layer of actively dividing cells with a pigment colour that has been altered due to a genetic mutation.

A classic example of genetic mutations creating variegated leaf colour is found in ivy. The ivy family demonstrates many different combinations of colours: green and white, yellow and green, red and green, and so on. Each of these colours is in fact a different layer of meristem tissue where genetic mutations in horizontally dividing layers have switched on or off specific colour pigments.

To come back to our question: is there an 'ideal' combination of colours for us to look at? A particularly ingenious study by an Assistant Professor of Landscape Design, Mohamed Elsadek, and his colleagues at the University of Chiba in Japan used these varieties of the two-toned ivy leaves to see if they could suggest an answer.[11]

The common or 'English' ivy (*Hedera helix*) is a species that, while having leaves all the same shape and size, includes a number of hybrid varieties with different coloured patterning. Some have wonderful descriptive names such as 'Goldchild' (yellow-green), 'Light Finger' (bright green), 'Glacier' (white-green), 'Pittsburgh Green' (dark green), and 'Pittsburgh Red' (orange-red).

In Elsadek's study, participants were asked to view five plant trays, in a randomly assigned order, with each tray containing a different variety of two-toned ivy. During the experiment brain scanning was carried out to detect neural activity, and two measurements of eye movements were taken, using a piece of equipment called an eye mark recorder, which measures both eye fixation-rates and small involuntary eye movements. These are both useful measures. The length of eye fixation, for example, has been shown to be associated with the amount of attention engaged when looking at something. In contrast, small involuntary eye movements (known as microsaccades) are related to aspects of vision associated with perception, attention and working memory.[12] In one experiment, when participants viewed a number of different images including a 'Where's Wally' picture, a natural scene, a picture puzzle and a blank screen, there were significantly increased microsaccades when scanning the natural scenes, suggesting that looking at nature can invoke greater attention (or at least more than looking for Wally).[13] Participants also filled out a questionnaire recording self-reported emotions after looking at each tray.

Results showed clearly that some two-tone colour combinations are better for us than others. In particular green-yellow and bright green ivy leaf varieties have the most positive outcomes, including enhanced neural activity in areas of the brain associated with a more relaxed and calm state, and longer eye-fixations and more microsaccades, indicating greater focus and attention.[14] And these two-colour combinations also gained the most positive responses in the questionnaires, with the words used to describe participants' feelings after viewing them including 'calm', 'stable', 'beautiful' and 'active'.

What I also found interesting was the conclusion that red leaves appeared to have the opposite, negative effect. Seeing these coloured leaves led to responses described as 'dark' and invoking feelings of tension. I think I might remove that red poinsettia on my desk.

The researchers concluded from this study that plants with green-yellow and bright green leaves should be incorporated into our living environments to induce calmness and to create feelings of cheerfulness and greater attention, a finding we could all carry into our daily lives.

But does our preference for these colours vary according to our cultural background? Other experiments, not specifically related to plants, have found that there are sometimes strong cultural differences in our colour preferences. Is the same true when looking at colours of plant leaves, and if so, does this preference influence the types of outcomes?

To address this Elsadek and his team repeated the ivy leaf experiment, but this time they involved forty participants, all young men, half of whom were from Japan and the other half from Egypt.[15] What emerged was evidence that while greens still elicited positive results, there were clear cultural differences. Whereas for the Egyptian participants bright green and green-yellow stimulated neural activity indicating enhanced calmness and feelings of cheerfulness, in the Japanese students it was dark green and green-white plants that invoked these positive responses. Although this is a very small sample size and only involved two cultures, this is an interesting result that warrants further research – especially if coloured foliage plants are used to help improve well-being in offices and homes.

Interestingly, in both groups red and orange colours invoked feelings of tension and anger, replicating the findings of many other studies.

But for me there is something here that doesn't quite add up. I began this chapter by recognising the universal appeal of the colours of a forest in autumn. But, if we have such a strong dislike of reds and oranges, why do people flock in their millions to see exactly these colours setting woods and trees ablaze all across the world? This made me start to wonder whether our preference for colour is fixed or whether in fact it is transient and changes according to season. Is green always best? Is it really time to bin the poinsettias?

The autumnal spectacle of leaf colour changing from green to orange and then red and brown occurs just before deciduous plants drop their leaves in response to a variety of external stimuli including lowering daily light levels, winter cooling (in temperate and boreal regions) and/or dry seasons (in tropical and sub-tropical regions).

The plants lose their leaves at these times in order to conserve water and energy during weather conditions that are not optimal for photosynthesis. This process of leaf loss is called leaf abscission, from the Latin words '*ab*' meaning 'away', and '*scindere*' meaning 'to split/cut'. Abscission takes place in a specific layer of cells where the leaf stalk joins the stem. This layer, called the abscission zone, is formed during the development of the leaf, and allows the flow of the growth hormone, auxin, into the leaf.

When it gets drier and/or colder, however, the flow of auxin becomes greatly reduced and the abscission zone becomes sensitive to another hormone called ethylene. Increased ethylene causes the build-up of enzymes which degrade the cell walls in the abscission zone, causing the leaf to break off from the branch.

By the time leaf abscission takes place, leaves are normally brown and dead (senesced). The brown colouration is due to the presence of tannin compounds and residual colour pigments in the dead leaf cells. It's the last stage of a dramatic leaf colour change: green, orange, red, brown. These autumnal colour changes are seen throughout the world but are perhaps most spectacular and celebrated in the temperate deciduous forests of New England in the north-eastern USA, and the beech forests of Patagonia and Japan. They are due to the presence of carotenoid pigments (which, as mentioned earlier, reflect orange-yellow colours back to us) and anthocyanin pigments (which reflect red-purple colours) in the leaves. Even though carotenoid pigments are present in leaves all the time, their colour is usually masked by the effect of the green-reflecting chlorophyll pigments. The reason we start to see them in autumn is that when there is a lowering of light and/or temperature, the chlorophyll (green) pigments in the leaves break down into colourless metabolites, and as a result the carotenoid (orange-yellow) pigments become more apparent. The red-purple colours are, however, due to a different process. The anthocyanin pigments, which give these characteristic colours, are newly generated in leaves shortly before leaf fall.[16]

So, we know why the wonderful shifting palette of green, yellow, orange, red, purple and brown is seasonally dependent, but what about our like/dislike of these colours? An experiment carried out by research psychologists Karen Schloss and Isobel Heck of the University of Wisconsin in 2017 certainly appears to suggest that they may also change with the seasons. When they asked a group of participants to rate their preferences for colours on a computer screen once a week over an eleven-week period spanning the autumn leaf fall between September and December, what emerged was a clearly increasing preference for red, yellow and orange colours during the weeks that the main fall was occurring, then tapering off again when winter set in after the fall (resulting in a U-shaped curve on the graph).[17]

Our likes and dislikes of leaf colours therefore appear to change with the seasons. Interestingly, there is also evidence emerging to suggest that there may be more physiological or psychological benefits to be gained from viewing red and orange foliage, compared to green, for certain groups of individuals. For example, one experiment that assessed children's perceived restoration potential when viewing different scenes of coloured foliage in their school playground showed that it was seeing trees with orange leaves, rather than green, which gave the greatest enhancement in restorative potential.[18] This curious result certainly needs more investigation, not least to understand if and how this changes over time and seasons, and, importantly, which species of trees should be planted around educational establishments. A second experiment involving patients with schizophrenia showed that when seeing orange and red foliage colours compared to green, their emotional arousal was significantly greater and more positive compared to when viewing green leaves.[19] Again, if this result is more widely replicated, it has important implications for choice of trees in healing gardens for patients suffering from conditions of this kind.

The emerging scientific evidence therefore is that green is good for us, and not just in what we eat. Seeing green leaves will make us calmer, happier, more focused and creative. But, perhaps surprisingly, in some respects foliage with more than one colour might be even better for us. Green–yellow variegated leaves seem to provide the best psychological and physiological outcomes, at least for some cultures. However, when autumn comes, we appear to switch sides and prefer yellows, oranges and reds – although we don't really know why, or whether this shift of allegiance is associated with any physiological or psychological changes. But it does seem that seeing red and orange leaves could potentially provide more psychological restoration and positive emotions among those with psychological disorders, and even children, than looking at green alone.

It's one of those findings which, when pointed out to you, you feel you already know it. We enjoy the colours of nature. They make us feel better. Why else do we flock to them for our holidays, and why do songwriters use 'those autumn leaves of red and gold' to summon up a certain kind of pleasantly indulgent melancholy? I know they have this effect on me. Memories of that road trip through the colours of New York stay with me, in my mind's eye and in treasured photos on my desk. It is reassuring to know that science is beginning to confirm that our instincts are right.

3

Flower Power

Last year, for the first time in many years, I visited the Chelsea Flower Show.

It was an enormous joy to wander once more along the gravel paths and between the colourful and varied gardens on display, enjoying the ingenuity of the themed and pop-up gardens and chatting to their creators, smelling the heady scents of the flowers and soaking up the passion and enthusiasm for weird and wonderful plants. The event has been running for over 100 years (with the inevitable break during Covid). Royalty and VIPs attend. Pictures of the show grace the front pages of our daily newspapers. Flowers, it seems, are as much a part of our English summer as cricket and cream teas.

It is also highly competitive. Growers compete for the coveted Royal Horticultural Society medals, and winners celebrate as if they'd just come first in the Flower Olympics. One of my proudest moments was when Kew won Gold at the 2017 show for our stand based around the second iteration of our horizon-scanning review of the status and condition of plant life across the world, and how this is changing over time, 'State Of The World's Plants'.[1]

Our display area was small, probably around twenty square metres (twenty-four square yards), yet somehow we managed to squeeze into this tiny space examples of the rarest and smallest plants in the world (such as the Rwandan water lily), conservation successes, extraordinary plants of Madagascar and plants that live in the most extreme environments. I can take no credit for the garden itself – this was thanks to the superb horticultural team at Kew who had spent months on the design, nurture of seedlings and planting. But the result was magnificent. It was like a dolls-house version of all the important and interesting things that we really need to know about the state of the world's plants. As one of my Malagasy colleagues, Dr Herizo Andrianandrasana, commented at the time, 'When people learn that 83 per cent of Madagascar's 11,138 native species of vascular plant occur nowhere else on earth, such as 84 per cent of Madagascar's thirty-seven native wild species of yam, we're not just giving people something unusual to look at: they are seeing biodiversity close up.'

Another impressive thing about the Chelsea Flower Show is the huge crowd of visitors who come to see the flowers. Flowers are a global attraction. People flock to see flowering plant displays in public gardens, parks and country estates all over the world. I watched this happening every day from my window when I worked at Kew Gardens and see it still in the Botanic Gardens and University Parks here in Oxford; like pollinating insects, we seem to be attracted to blowsy, colourful blooms in herbaceous borders.

Nor would it appear that our connection with the visual stimulus of flowers is just about neatly arranged blocks of bright colours, as Chelsea proves. This year, 2023, a

Gold medallist was Lindum's Wildflower Turf, containing twenty-seven species of native UK wildflowers, perennials and herbs that will support a range of pollinators and insects, using peat-free, recycled compost and requiring minimal maintenance: beautiful, soothing, but a million miles from the manicured, daisy-free lawns of more formal herbaceous borders and public gardens.

Seeing flowers, then, appears to do something important for us as humans. This chapter sets out to find out what it is and how it works.

We've certainly known about the beneficial and enjoyable effects of being surrounded by colourful flowers for a very long time. Writing in 1949, the historian of gardening J. W. Morton tells us that 'Egyptian tomb paintings from around 1500 BCE provide some of the earliest physical evidence of ornamental horticulture and landscape design; depicting lotus ponds surrounded by symmetrical rows of acacias and palms.'[2] The Hanging Gardens of Babylon were one of the Seven Wonders of the Ancient World. Rich Romans placed formal statues in their estates bordered with hedges and vines and ornamented with acanthus, cornflowers, crocus, cyclamen, hyacinth, iris, ivy, lavender, lilies, myrtle, narcissus, poppy, rosemary and violets. The Middle Ages developed the 'walled garden', principally for producing food and medicinal herbs, but also for growing plants with symbolic functions in decorating church and home at various seasons of the year and, later, for display and enjoyment. Renaissance gardens set flowers in the context of architectural and geometrical features such as 'knot gardens' and elaborate fountains. Ordinary people grew flowers, too, with the growth of the cottage garden, combining pleasure and practicality in a private acre stocked with herbs, fruit trees and flowering plants to support the family beehive. In the eighteenth century, the formal, classical 'French' style gave way to naturalistic landscape designs.

Herbaceous borders as we know them today, featuring a profusion of flowers of different shapes and sizes, became a feature of gardens in the western world from around the late nineteenth century. In 1883, William Robinson's seminal book *The English Flower Garden* scorned the use of the conservatory and hothouse in favour of a more naturalistic approach. Architects and designers such as William Morris, C.F.A. Voysey and Edwin Lutyens integrated house into garden and garden into house, 'as if Spring had come all of a sudden', as a colleague of Voysey's remarked. Most influential of all was Lutyens' regular collaborator, the gardener and garden designer Gertrude Jekyll, who created some 400 gardens and wrote copiously on the subject of garden design, including over 1,000 articles for magazines and newspapers. Her distinctive painterly approach to combinations of colour can be admired today in gardens like Sissinghurst Castle in Kent, created by her friend Vita Sackville-West.

As well as enjoying colourful flowers in our gardens, we cut them and bring them indoors: a habit that also has deep historical roots. As one commentator records, 'A 2,000-year-old funerary garland found at Egypt's Hawara burial site contains chrysanthemum flowers, twigs of sweet marjoram and hibiscus petals.' Roman mosaics show young women wearing wreaths of cut flowers in their hair in honour of the goddess Flora. However, it was the Dutch who launched the modern flower trade, exploiting and developing international routes to import exotic species; the collapse of the market caused by Tulipmania in the 1630s is still Lesson One in economics textbooks and courses today (though apparently not one we have fully learned). The Victorians favoured large, elaborate bouquets, and followed folklore and Shakespeare in ascribing meaning and features to particular species, as in Kate Greenaway's 1884 book *Language of Flowers*: forget-me-not for true love, flytrap for deceit, French marigold for jealousy.

Today, we still use our affinity for cut flowers to symbolise aspects of custom and routine, reaching for particular colours and varieties at Christmas and Easter, on birthdays and at weddings. Funeral directors report that when a notice requests 'No Flowers', people bring and send them anyway, as if they answer some deep instinct, or carry an emotional message on our behalf.

And, of course, the popularity of cut flowers makes them big business, not least because so many of them are grown far from where they are sold, travelling across borders to bring the colours of one country and climate to another: in 2022 the global cut flower market was estimated to be worth $35.6 billion (£28 billion).

But to the investigation in hand. Does looking at flowers have measurable health benefits in addition to those in the previous chapter that come from seeing green? Two simple experiments made me realise that when we see flowers, there is far more going on than meets the eye.

In the first experiment, a team of psychologists led by Professor Jeannette Haviland-Jones of the State University of New Jersey measured facial responses of individuals receiving a gift of a bunch of flowers, a pen or another non-flower gift.[3] They found that the individuals' responses were significantly different. The flowers elicited a 'Duchenne smile' within five seconds of receiving the gift (this is a smile, often referred to as a 'true smile', that engages muscles around our mouth and eyes and is thought to be related to positive changes in brain chemistry and various psychophysiological indices). The pen or other gift didn't elicit the same kind of response.

In the second experiment, a team of scientists from the Centre for Environment, Health and Field Sciences in Chiba University examined the effects on office workers of having a vase of flowers on their desks.[4] Remarkably they found that exposure to unscented pink roses (without leaves) for just four minutes resulted in clear evidence of physiological and psychological calming, compared to when they sat at desks with no flowers. The participants also reported, in a self-assessment questionnaire, that they felt more comfortable and relaxed when the vase of roses was present.[5]

These preliminary studies hint that seeing flowers can trigger positive physiological and psychological health outcomes. But is this the case with all flowers or are there particular shapes and colours of flowers that are better for bringing about these sorts of outcomes? And do these flowers need to be real, or can we gain the same benefits from plastic versions? I say this because if the shelves in large homeware stores are anything to go by, the production of artificial flowers certainly seems to be blooming (forgive the pun!).

Flowers represent a colourful evolutionary success story. Today, around 96 per cent of the world's flora is composed of flowering plants, but this has not always been the case. In fact, flowering plants are the most recent group of plants to evolve, first appearing in the fossil record around 130 million years ago before arriving at their present diversity and ubiquity something like seventy million years ago.[6] Before this, the vegetation on the planet looked very different. It was dominated by groups of plants such as the gymnosperms (which include conifers and cycads), ferns and horsetails, and lycopods. The often-cited statement that the earliest large herbivorous dinosaurs on the Earth, such as sauropods and stegosaurus, would never have seen a flower or walked on grass (grasses are also flowering plants), is broadly correct.

The evolution of flowers was an incredibly important innovation. This is because their multiple colours, patterns and shapes provided many different ways to become successfully fertilised (wind pollination, animal pollination) and reproduce (sexual and asexual reproduction). This enabled highly successful and often fast colonisation of a large variety of different environments, and flowering plants (angiosperms) quickly outcompeted the gymnosperms, ferns, horsetails and lycopods in most landscapes. Within a matter of twenty to thirty million years after first appearing in the fossil record they became the dominant plants in many regions in the world.

The variety of flower shape, colour and size around the globe is something to behold. For example, the smallest flowers in the world are less than one millimetre (0.04 inches) in diameter, white and belong to an aquatic species of duckweed (*Wolffia microscopia*). By contrast the largest are over one metre (forty inches) in diameter, bright red with orange-white spots and belong to the giant corpse flower (*Rafflesia arnoldii*) which gets its common name from its rather unpleasant scent, apparently smelling like rotting human flesh.

The huge variation in flower sizes is determined by genetic processes influencing the rates of cell division and cell expansion in the developing flower.[7] Another genetically determined aspect is the shape of the petals. In this case, the genes influence differential rates of growth in the petal tissue. For example, in the development of the characteristic trumpet-shaped flowers seen in species such as Petunia (*Petunia* spp.), when the flowers start to grow, cell division and elongation occurs evenly throughout the petal and the long tube is developed. However, as the flower comes close to its maximum size, a slowdown in the division of cells begins first at the base of the petal. There is then a slowdown in the other dividing cells from base to tip, so that the cells at the tip are still dividing relatively fast compared to those at the base. This process of differential cell growth rates in the petal tissue results in the top part growing faster, forming the large flowery trumpet-like head emerging from a long tube-like neck.

Curvature of the petal is also genetically controlled. In lily flowers (*Lilium* spp.), for example, the characteristic curved petals are the result of a faster rate of cell division at the margins of the petal relative to those in the centre.

However, it is not just the shape and curvature of the petals that distinguishes between different flowers, but also the arrangement of flower parts (petals, sepals, stamens and carpels).

The names and arrangement of these organs is something most of us learn at school – over and over again. Drawing a cross-section of a flower showing its reproductive structures is possibly one of the most boring things a reluctant schoolchild ever had to do. Children in the UK are also made to learn and re-learn this up to four times during their education, and I am firmly of the belief that this is one of the reasons why so many are permanently put off studying plant biology to degree level; we certainly don't do this repetitive learning of the cross-section of any other organism, like a dog or a snail, for example.

But I digress – the symmetrical or otherwise arrangement of the reproductive parts of a flower and petals are as a consequence of differential gene expression, resulting in structures that tend to be either radially symmetrical with many lines of symmetry, such as Black-eyed Susan daisies (*Rudbeckia hirta*), or have a single plane of symmetry, such as those in the pea family Fabaceae, for example the sweet pea (*Lathyrus latifolius*). The latter are known as bilateral or zygomorphic. There are also some flower shapes that have a symmetry that is contorted to the left or right, including some aquatic plants, but these are much rarer than symmetrical and zygomorphic forms.

In addition to size, shape and arrangement of reproductive organs, the most distinguishing feature between different flowers is colour. And, similar to leaves, flower colour is as a result of pigments in the petal tissues, micro-structural features on the surface of the petal and internal cell arrangements.[8]

The most common pigments determining petal colour fall into four main groups: flavonoids, carotenoids, betalains and

chlorophylls. The flavonoids, which reflect back a number
of different colours in the wavelength, are responsible for
ivory and cream-coloured petals. Carotenoids are mainly
responsible for yellow and orange colours, including bright
yellow sunflowers (*Helianthus annuus*). Betalains provide
the red and pink colours for one specific groups of plants
called the Caryophyllales which includes cacti, carnations,
amaranths, ice plants, beets, the red-purple varieties of
Bougainvillea and pink carnations. And finally, some petals
contain the green pigment chlorophyll. Even though this
is much less common in petals than leaves, a number of
plant species have green flowers, including for example the
green hellebore (*Helleborus viridis*).

As an aside, an interesting fact that I came across during
this research is that the colour they reflect can be affected
by the pH value and the presence of metal ions in the soil.[9]
Blue hydrangeas (*Hydrangea macrophylla*), for example, are
blue in colour if there is aluminium in the soil and it is
acidic, but reddish-pink in alkaline soils. This is because
the metal ions interact with the plant pigments to create
molecules that have spectral properties that absorb different
wavelengths.

Microstructural features in the petals can also influence
flower colour. In petals, these nano-scale structures
include cones and ridges made of transparent material.
These shaped features change the angle of reflected light,
often splitting the wavelength so that the full spectrum
of rainbow colours is displayed in an iridescent sheen.[10]
This effect is more pronounced on dark-coloured flowers
including, for example, the 'Queen of the Night' tulip,
which has iridescent colours on a purple background.

As in leaves, internal micro-structural features are also responsible for flower colour and surface. One, which most of us will have encountered at some point in our childhood, results in the shiny yellow surface of the petal of the common buttercup (*Ranunculus repens*), which reflects the colour onto our chins if we hold the flower under them. The yellow colour is caused by an abundance of carotenoid pigments that absorb the blue-green light and reflect yellow light. The shiny effect, however, is as a result of two layers of cells in the petal that produce a double-mirror-like effect when light hits them.[11]

Another factor affecting colour and combination of colours in flowers may come as a slightly unwelcome surprise: disease. As with leaves, genetic mutations and diseases in plants can affect flower colour and patterning. Many of us will probably be aware of the browning of petals, spots, rusts and the unattractive curling of flowers when infected with a fungal, bacterial or viral infection. However, a genetic mutation, or infection with a bacteria or virus does not always result in the death of the plant. And we may not be aware that some of the most sought-after ornamental plants have their beautiful colour combinations on their petals because of past or current viral infections.

There are a number of viruses known to cause flower breaking, the term given to variegated colour patterns on petals due to the irregular distributions of pigments. This includes, for example, the mosaic patterns on the leaves of the flowering maple (*Abutilon pictum*) when infected with the abutilon mosaic virus (*Begomovirus*). Probably one of the most famous, however, is the Potyvirus, which causes the striking flame- or feather-like patterns on red and yellow striped tulips. This rare and striking effect made them hugely prized in seventeenth-century Holland. They are often seen in paintings by Rembrandt and others, and indeed are sometimes known as Rembrandt's tulips. Inflated prices for these prized polychromatic blooms contributed to the collapse of the Dutch economy caused by Tulipmania. This colour variegation occurs because virus-infected cells in the growing tissue (in the meristem) are unable to produce red coloured pigments (anthocyanin). As the tulip petals grow by cell division, those cells that divide without anthocyanin form coloured yellow streaks up the petal. It should be noted, however, that this virus pattern was not reliably transferred to subsequent generations and the vast majority of striped tulips that we see presently are as a result of later genetic modification of these plants by plant breeders.

With so much variation in flowers, returning to the question posed at the beginning of the chapter, do we have a preference for particular shapes and colours? And if so, are the ones we instinctively prefer, and give to other people as gifts, the most beneficial in terms of their health outcomes?

There certainly appears to be a pattern in terms of the colour of flowers that we give as gifts. When researchers looked at US consumer transactions for monthly purchasing of cut flowers between 1992 and 2005 across forty-nine US states, they found that red-bronze flowers were the most purchased, whereas yellow flowers were the least favoured.[12] This selection choice, however, was also influenced by the occasion for buying the flowers. It would appear that people in the US, at least, tend to buy red-bronze flowers for an anniversary, and peach-pink flowers for Mother's Day (though, as discussed below, more work remains to be done on the extent to which these choices are culturally determined or somehow psychologically innate).[13]

But what happens when we are not selecting flowers for a particular occasion? Do we have an automatic preference for particular shapes and colours of flowers? Although few studies have addressed this question to date, an experiment in 2016 by scientists Martin Hůla and Jaroslav Flegr from Charles University in the Czech Republic revealed some interesting, and, for me, somewhat surprising findings.[14]

Fifty-two different flower types were chosen for this study to illustrate a range of different colours, symmetry and curvature of the outline contours (angularity). All were native to the Czech Republic but not commonplace, to ensure that selection by participants was not unduly biased by familiarity. These fifty-two flowers were presented in an online survey of over 2,000 participants from the Czech Republic with ages ranging between twelve and seventy-four years. Each participant was asked to view the photos and rate them according to their beauty, complexity and how representative they thought it was of a 'typical flower'. The order of the flower photos was also randomised so that no one person saw them in the same order.

What they found was that, regardless of age and gender of the participants, the flowers chosen as most beautiful were blue, followed by purple, then pink. It is worth noting here that there were no green flowers in this experiment, but that green is in the same part of the colour wavelength spectrum as blue and purple. In comparison, the colour white, which is at the other end of the colour spectrum, had no significant effect, and yellow was rated as the least attractive flower colour. However, most interesting was the finding that the strongest feature influencing the perception of beauty was not colour but shape. Those flowers with the highest preference ratings were symmetrical in shape of petals and reproductive organs, and with a mid-level of complexity.

While these findings suggest that we might have an affinity to certain types of flowers, I want to add in a note of caution here: this is a single study (although with a large number of participants) and based on the population of one country. It is entirely possible therefore that the findings would be different with other cultural groups. What also worries me slightly is the fact that the 'preferred criteria' to emerge from this study represent the total opposite to flowers in the Orchidaceae family, which have symmetry in one plane, rounded-petal edges and are often white or yellow in colour. Yet orchids are possibly one of the most widely cherished and purchased flowers for display in homes, offices and glasshouses throughout the world, and have been for over 200 years. Early plant hunters travelled the world to find new weird and wonderful varieties.[15] Perhaps in this instance, rarity and exoticism trumps the usual preferences for shape and colour.

What these preference experiments also don't tell us is whether seeing different flower shapes and colours has any measurable impact on our physical and mental well-being. Given what we know about our preferences with green and coloured leaves, is the same also true for colours in flowers?

In order to address this question, research scientists made clever use of an approach similar to the ivy experiment described in Chapter 2, choosing a plant species that produces flowers with many varieties of colour, but broadly consistent in terms of size and shape.[16] The species they selected was the succulent plant genus *Kalanchoe*, often known as widow's-thrill, which has white, yellow, pink and red flowers. The common houseplant *Epipremnum aureum* (devil's ivy) was used as a control since it has evergreen leaves and rarely flowers, and could thus provide a direct comparison of response between seeing green leaves and seeing flowers of many different colours.

Participants were each asked to view five boxes containing examples of one of these two species for three minutes each, with a two-minute break between them, in a randomly assigned order. While doing so, brain activity was assessed (using EEG) in four areas of the brain: the prefrontal, frontal, parietal and occipital lobes. These different areas of the brain are thought to be related to different functions including creativity, intellectual capacity, verbal processing and visual abilities. After each viewing the participants also filled in a questionnaire to assess their emotional responses to the different plant colour stimuli.

All the plants, whatever the colour or shape, correlated with some enhanced brain activity and emotional response compared to the baseline measurements, once again confirming that seeing any vegetation is better than none at all. However, clear differences emerged with the colour of the flowers. The participants' brain functions were significantly more active in regions associated with improved concentration, creativity and attention, and they also reported feeling more cheerful and positive when they viewed the devil's ivy plant with its predominantly green leaves. The other colour to demonstrate this enhanced impact was yellow. Interestingly, this is the exact opposite to the Czech study mentioned above, which tested preference and emotional response rather than analysing effects on brain functionality: we may *think* we prefer blue/green flowers and not yellow; but seeing yellow may make us more creative and work better.

These preliminary results, which have since been repeated in a number of similar studies, indicate that, as with leaves (see Chapter 1), green and yellow should be the go-to colours of choice for flowers in our homes and offices.[17] These two colours appear to trigger the most positive physiological and psychological responses when we look at them.[18] In comparison, white flowers don't seem to be very good at doing these things.[19]

Colour, then, matters. What we see when we interact with nature has measurable effects on our physical and mental well-being. The colours, shades and combinations of colours displayed by both leaves and flowers play an important part in that.

But there's a new kid on the block when it comes to decorating our internal and external spaces with vegetation: fake plants. Fake plants seem to be growing in popularity in offices and homes and the market in artificial plants is rapidly increasing. A recent report estimated that it is projected to reach $780.3 million (£618 million) by 2028.[20] Many varieties of material are used to make artificial flowers, and some of them are remarkably realistic – especially those made from polyester, with these often appearing in the most unexpected places. Several years ago, I found myself in the offices of the UK government's Department of the

Environment and Rural Affairs (DEFRA), which works on UK and international policies to conserve and enhance nature. Seeing a wonderful flowering plant on the table in the meeting room, I went up closer to see what species it was, only to find when touching its leaves that it was made of polyester. Of all the places I did not expect to find fake plants, DEFRA was top of the list! Leaving aside the environmental impacts of making plants out of synthetic materials such as polyester and plastics, it made me wonder whether it matters if they are real or not for the health benefits that they confer? Is viewing these 'fake' versions as effective in reducing stress and improving our mood – or do we need the real thing?

Several studies have addressed this question, including a neat experiment from 2015 in which high school student participants were asked to view, for three minutes, either a planter containing fresh yellow pansies (*Viola* x *wittrockiana*) or 'pansies' identical in colour, size and markings in an identical container, but this time made of polyester.[21] Then, after a break, they were presented with the other planter (the order of viewing them was random to reduce any bias in terms of timing), unaware of which was which. As with other experiments described in this book, physiological stress measures (heart-rate variability and pulse rate) were taken during the process of viewing and questionnaires to subjectively evaluate their psychological state were filled out afterwards.

Surprisingly significant differences emerged. Visual stimulation from real flowers resulted in a significant decrease in physiological stress compared to looking at the fake pansies. The students also stated that they were more comfortable and relaxed when viewing the real pansies compared to artificial. I found other studies showing similar results, suggesting that the answer to the question 'will artificial versions of flowers do?' is probably 'no' – even though fake plants might look nice, they do not appear to confer the same stress reduction and mood improvements as the real thing.

So far my focus has been on examining the responses to single-colour cut flowers and to colours associated with typical houseplants. But in natural settings and semi-natural environments, such as public spaces, botanic gardens and even our own back gardens, of course, we rarely look at a single colour, shape or type of flower, but a mixture of these things in infinite and constantly changing combinations. So, what happens when we look at colourful flowering borders of the type we encounter in botanic gardens and places like the Chelsea Flower Show? When we see more colours and variety, do the health benefits increase? This question is particularly pertinent for planning city parks and urban green spaces where there is often a tendency to prioritise large expanses of mown grass for recreation. Most parks will also have trees and some shrubs around the edges, but colourful herbaceous flowering borders and wildflower meadows are often absent, not least because maintenance requires resources.

I also wondered whether we should be focusing on diversity of colour or species type. For example, as a botanist, I find a natural chalk grassland a wonderful environment to visit, due to the huge variety of herbaceous grassland species. The problem is, to someone else, this will look like a vast expanse of boring green grass, since most of these species are the same colour, and the flowers that grow on chalk grassland tend to be small and difficult to see from any distance.

I was, therefore, intrigued to come across the results of several studies that have started to address these questions, both in the UK and the US. These are revealing some important policy-relevant findings, but possibly not ones that will cheer enthusiasts for chalk grassland like me. It would appear, on a landscape, the more blowsy the colours and varieties we see, the better the outcomes for our health and well-being.

To take one example, Helen Hoyle and colleagues from the University of Sheffield selected thirty UK public gardens and categorised them according to their percentage of woodland, shrub and herbaceous planting and flower cover.[22] They then surveyed 1,411 members of the public who visited these gardens and asked them to complete a site-based questionnaire designed to capture their perceptions of the gardens' aesthetic qualities and restorative effect, and the perceived biodiversity value of the gardens. Clear results emerged. Public gardens with colourful planting and bright flowers came top for aesthetic preference and were typically rated as extremely attractive and stimulating, particularly when flower cover accounted for more than 27 per cent of the garden.

Also of interest in this study was the finding that while colour appeared to provide the 'wow' factor, subtle green colours were rated as more conducive to quiet reflection and inducing a restorative effect. This very much builds on the findings discussed previously, suggesting that both colourful flowers and green foliage appear to be important for enhancing mental well-being.

On the other side of the Atlantic similar findings were also found by Rose Graves and colleagues from the University of Wisconsin–Madison. They surveyed 293 visitors to the Appalachian forests during the summer of 2015 and asked them to select their favourite images of wildflower communities. These featured a mixture of different combinations of species richness, abundance, colour diversity and charismatic species. They found similar results to Hoyle's UK experiment. Aesthetic preference increased when they showed more abundant flowers and greater colour diversity. Also, these aesthetic preferences were consistent across different demographic groups and appear to be unaffected by a knowledge of local flora.[23]

The take-home message from these two studies, therefore, is that there is a positive relationship between what we see, what we say we like, and what is good for us. In all cases, an abundance of colour comes top.[24] However, the number of studies examining the impacts of higher biodiversity (colour or species diversity) on our well-being is currently very small, and they rely almost entirely upon self-reported assessments, so these results should be treated as preliminary. In fact, I came across no studies that have attempted to understand what happens to us physiologically when we view herbaceous borders with colourful floral displays compared to grasslands. This seems an important knowledge gap to fill, given its relevance for management of public green spaces across the world.

Another point worth flagging up here is that when researching the effect of colourful planting schemes on us, we also need to be mindful of the potential impact of cultural differences. A study that illustrates this point well is one that asked the same questions about preference for biodiverse planting in parks, but this time in Beijing, China. The findings were very different from those from the UK and US. Of the 227 Chinese students and professionals asked to rate their aesthetic preference for photos of wildflower meadows in comparison to highly ordered flowerbeds in Beijing's urban parks, the wildflower meadows, containing multiple different brightly coloured flowers, had the lowest satisfaction rating.[25] Why? In the participants' responses to the questionnaire, it was apparent that many viewed wildflower meadows as 'unkempt' and instead preferred the controlled and well-arranged flowerbeds between mown grassy lawns.

This chapter began with a pleasant stroll around the colourful exhibits at the Chelsea Flower Show. Chelsea provides a striking example of our strong desire to see flowers in all shapes and sizes. It is becoming clear from the scientific evidence that, when we do so, they confer a host of health benefits. Seeing flowers of different colours and shapes affects how we feel and how we work, and mostly for the better. We clearly need them in our day-to-day environment. But, as so often, anomalies remain. Studies to date show some apparent contradictions in exactly which colours work best in achieving particular outcomes in particular contexts, including cultural. We still need more work to understand which colours and varieties to choose.

But we can and should change our behaviour and our environment to incorporate the flowery benefits that we do already know about. We should make visits to parks and other landscapes with colourful flowers a priority. Use the colours of flowers in your home, school and workplace. Insist that window boxes, pocket parks and patches of wildflowers are part of the urban environment where you live. And make an annual pilgrimage to Chelsea or your nearest equivalent. But book early: people like flowers.

4

The Sweet Smell of Success:
Protective Plant Perfumes

Recently, I found myself climbing the winding wood-panelled staircase of a handsome Georgian shop at 89 Jermyn Street, in the heart of St James's, one of the oldest districts of central London. The dark stairs opened into a large, light room furnished with polished tables and hung with portraits. I was greeted by Edward Bodenham, who bore a striking resemblance to many of the faces in the paintings and photographs around him, as well he might: these were his ancestors, nine generations of the Bodenham and Floris families. This has been the headquarters of his family firm since 1730. The business does today what it has done on the same site for almost 300 years: make and sell perfume, using natural ingredients from a wide and sometimes surprising range of sources and places.

Edward took me through the fascinating history of his company and family: the receipts recording sales to Winston Churchill and Marilyn Monroe, the mentions of his products in no fewer than three of the James Bond novels by regular customer Ian Fleming, the marriage of Mary Anne Floris and James Bodenham in 1870, the letter from Florence Nightingale recording her thanks for the 'beautiful sweet-smelling nosegays', the royal warrant of

1820, and the letters home of Robert Floris to his parents, founder Juan Famenias Floris and his wife Elizabeth, as he sailed the world searching for ingredients in the 1700s. He also talked me through the basics of choosing different scents for perfumes and their properties for selection – including the use of so-called base notes.

Base notes have a chemical make-up which means that, when mixed with other scents, they enhance the attractive floral top notes. Surprisingly, these base notes are not always that nice to smell by themselves and can come from some less than desirable sources. For example, the smell civet comes from the soft, paste-like glandular secretion from underneath the striped tails of civet cats. Musk is extracted from the gland located near the tail of male musk deer – an unpleasant smell on its own but apparently much more agreeable when combined with other scents. Ambergris comes from digested squid beaks in whale poo. Who would have guessed beautifully smelling perfumes can contain these products? These animal-based smells are now usually created in the laboratory – but it wasn't that far back that the real animal versions were used. I didn't ask how they extracted them: too much information.

Not surprisingly, our relationship with the smells of nature goes back further even than Edward's illustrious forebears. There is, in fact, considerable early documentation recording the use of different plant smells for beautification, for rituals and for masking other less desirable odours such as decaying bodies. None more so than in ancient Egypt. In the mummification process, cinnamon, which is a scented spice obtained from the inner bark of several tree species in the plant genus *Cinnamomum*, was stuffed into the body cavity to provide a more lifelike appearance and to reduce the smell of the rotting flesh. The linens wrapped around the body were also applied with various plant scents infused in oil.

Archaeological exploration has also revealed that the ancient Egyptians mass-produced scents for use as fragrance. Excavations at Thumis, north of Cairo on the Nile Delta, found an area riddled with tiny glass perfume bottles and clay amphoras, dated to 300 BCE.[1] Chemical analysis of dried residue in these vessels revealed that they contained a mixture of scented plant material and olive oil. This included myrrh, a natural resin extracted from a thorny tree species *Commiphora myrrha*; cardamom, a scented spice made from the seeds of plants in the genera *Elettaria* and *Amomum*; and cinnamon. When this mixture was recreated in the laboratory it was found that the perfume has a musky smell and was much thicker and oilier than those we use now; I'm not sure how commercially viable this kind of recipe would be today.

What my brief foray into the origins of the perfume industry and its history confirmed to me is that we have a long-established impulse to surround ourselves with the more salubrious scents of nature. But what also emerges from history is that our ancestors spent considerable time examining the production and movement of different smells, how they were transmitted into our bodies, and their potential impacts on our health.

Some of the earliest writings on these topics came from the early philosophers Aristotle and Plato. Aristotle believed that smell required a medium for transmission – although he didn't elaborate what this medium might be. Plato, by contrast, believed smell was transmitted by fumes or vapours, stating his observation that 'smells always proceed from bodies that are damp, or putrefying, or liquefying, or evaporating'.[2] Medieval thinkers took sides: the twelfth-century monk William of St-Thierry believed that 'the fumes from odorous bodies, dissolved and mixed with the air, are drawn in through the openings of the nostrils ... [and] transmitted to the brain'. The seventeenth-century English scientist Robert Boyle firmly believed that smell must be conveyed by the transmission of some physical substance. Boyle called this physical matter 'magnetic steams', and noted, as all of us who have the pleasure to count dogs as members of our families have also noticed, that 'the steams [discernible by dogs] ... must be of an extreme, and scarce conceivable minuteness'.[3]

What Plato and Aristotle did agree on, however, was that medicinal and therapeutic powers were obtained from these plant odours. This was a theme that was very much in the mind of Carl Linnaeus, often referred to as the father of modern botany, when he started to question the medicinal role of different scents in the eighteenth century. One particularly noteworthy piece of work that attempted to classify different plant smells into types was *Dissertatio medica odores medicamentorum exhibens* (*Dissertation on the odours exhibited by different medicinal plants*), published in 1752 by Linnaeus and his student Andreas Wåhlin.[4] Wåhlin and Linnaeus divided plant odours into seven classes – some of which will be instantly recognisable to anyone reading them today: aromatic; fragrant; ambrosial (musky); hircine (goat-like); foul (repulsive); nauseating (disgusting); and alliaceous (garlicky). They are at pains to point out that their essay is not just an exercise in classifying the many thousands of smells emitted by plants, of which 'scarcely two are so similar in smell that no difference can be felt', but specifically to investigate the '*actio quidem rerum odoriferarum in corpus humanum*': 'the action of odoriferous things on the human body'.[5]

Besides being used because of their nice smell, scents have therefore long also been used for medicinal purposes – and not always because the smell itself was particularly pleasing. Many eighteenth- and nineteenth-century bodice-rippers, for example, feature the use of smelling salts to rouse the fainting heroine from a fit of the vapours. These foul-smelling salts were used to arouse consciousness because they release ammonia (NH_3) gas which irritates the membranes of the nose and lungs, and thereby triggers an inhalation reflex. This reflex alters the pattern of breathing, resulting in improved respiratory flow rates and possibly alertness. I was surprised to discover that it is still possible to buy a large variety of smelling salts online today.

So, what do we now know about what happens when we inhale different plant smells? Compared to our understanding of other senses, the science of smell has been something of a Cinderella subject. For example, a detailed understanding of the genes responsible for our ability to smell only emerged as recently as 2004.[6] This is decades behind our knowledge on the genetic code for our other senses such as sight. Recent advances have also demonstrated that, despite the oft-cited statement that we have a poor sense of smell, humans can in fact discriminate at least one *trillion* different smells.[7] Our sense of smell is apparently still not as good as that of dogs, but we certainly have a far more discerning nose than previously thought. This is thanks to around 400 olfactory receptors in our noses, sometimes referred to as smell receptors. These are proteins clustered in specialised cells in a small area at the back of our nasal cavity called the olfactory epithelium. When we sniff a scent, these receptors bind to the specific odour molecules inhaled, causing the olfactory receptor proteins to become stimulated. This action triggers nerve impulses which send information via electrical signals about the odour to our brain.[8]

The area of the brain triggered by the electrical smell signals is called the forebrain or olfactory bulb and can be found in the forward-most section of our brain, just above our nose. It is a complex part of the brain with over 400 distinct areas, each activated by a specific odour. From here information passes via electrical signals into another part of our brain called the olfactory cortex, and then on to other sections including the hippocampus, thalamus and frontal cortex. The movement of these electrical signals accounts for how our brains process and interpret information about smell, including intensity and odour memory.[9] In addition, and most relevant to our health, these signals also trigger other involuntary pathways (nervous, endocrine and psychological), which can lead to physiological and psychological changes when we smell certain scents. In many ways, these changes are the same as those that occur when we see a visual image. Our brains not only process information about what we are smelling; the act of smelling also triggers involuntary responses in our bodies resulting in both physical and mental changes.

However, an additional process, different from our reaction to the other senses, occurs when we smell something.

When we inhale smells, some of the odour molecules are absorbed via the membranes in our lungs and pass across into our bloodstream. From here they directly interact with various biochemical pathways, sometimes bringing about the sort of changes associated with taking a prescription drug, such as for a reduction in anxiety. A visual or aural stimulus doesn't do this. Smelling certain compounds therefore directly introduces something physical into our bloodstream in a way that sight and sound cannot.

The transfer of smell compounds into our blood really became clear to me when I came across a study looking at what happens when we walk in a scented coniferous forest. Kazuhiro Sumitomo and colleagues from Asahikawa Medical University in Hokkaido examined the profile of the bloods of a group of volunteers before and after they walked for sixty minutes in a scented cypress forest. This environment gets its characteristic 'pine-like' smell from the volatile organic compounds given out by many conifer trees, including cypress, called α-pinene. What they found was a large increase of α-pinene in the participants' blood after the walk; in effect what they were detecting was these scent molecules passing from the ambient air in the forests into the participants' bloodstreams, via their lungs.[10]

The fact that smelling certain scents not only triggers involuntary pathways in our bodies, bringing about physiological and psychological changes, but also can pass molecules into our blood and potentially impact biochemical pathways was a revelation to me.

To really understand the full significance of the impact of the smells of nature and in particular those from plants

Changes of VOC pinene in participants' blood after walking in a coniferous forest

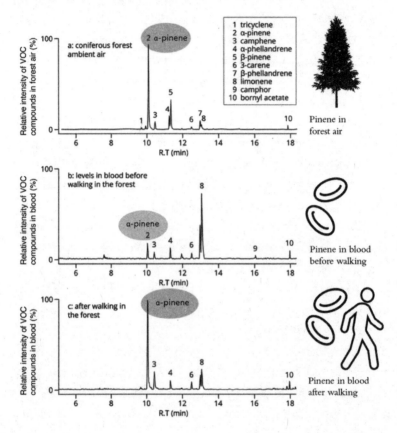

Source: K. Sumitomo et al.

on our health requires two more steps: first, what are the chemical compounds that make up plant smells; and second, is there any evidence that smelling these scents brings about health benefits and, if so, which particular plant scents are most effective?

If you ask people which part of a plant scents come from most people would probably say from the flowers. And this is partially correct. Many flower heads contain specialised scent-producing structures. Some also contain scent cells in the petal tissue. When you squeeze the petals of certain rose species, such as floribunda roses, between your fingers and a wonderful scent emerges, it's obvious where the smell comes from. Less well known is the fact that scent cells are also found in leaves, needles, leaf hairs, bark and even the stems of some trees. Hard lumps of sweet-scented resin, such as frankincense and myrrh for example, which were first used by the ancient Egyptians for their smell, are in fact the dried version of a sticky sap that is produced by specialised cells located in the stems of certain species of woody trees and shrubby plants. The sap is released in response to mechanical damage to the trunk caused by cutting or chewing, to protect the wound from further attack and decay.

The ingredients responsible for the scents emitted from plants are carbon-based compounds called volatile organic compounds. They are released from a plant as a gaseous cloud and evaporate easily at room temperature. More than 1,700 volatile organic compounds have been identified in different plant species in around ninety different plant families.

Usually, plant scents are made up of a combination of these different compounds with most common plant smells composed of between twenty and sixty different components.[11] This means that if totally different plant species have broadly the same concentrations of compounds, they will smell the same. For example, a volatile organic compound called coumarin is dominant in vanilla grass

(*Anthoxanthum odoratum*), tonka beans (*Dipteryx odorata*) and sweet clover (*Melilotus officinalis*), resulting in a similar smell coming from all three plants.

These organic carbon-based compounds are formed into carbon chains of varying lengths, shapes and complexity, and this is what creates the smell when it is released from the plant as a gas. For example, the description 'fresh' and 'green' often given to the smell associated with walking across a freshly cut lawn is due to the release of simple straight carbon chains of alcohols and aldehydes known as the green-leaf volatiles.[12]

The majority of the plant smells that we encounter on a daily basis are made up of far more complex structures, consisting of carbon chains that are kinked and twisted, and include a large number of different chemicals. Volatile organic compounds formed into these distinctive twisted and complex-structured compounds are known as terpenes, and are further classified by the number of carbon atoms they contain (e.g. sesquiterpenes, which have fifteen carbon atoms).

Terpenes are responsible for a number of well-known scents, including one that we probably smell every day without even thinking about it, called linalool. Linalool is present in over 200 plant species and 50 per cent of plant families, and its strong sweet 'flowery' smell is often commercially manufactured for use in household products from soaps and shampoos to air fresheners and polish. Linalool also forms the base note for many perfumes.

Examples of other well-known smells emerging from terpenes include the scents of pine (α-pinene, ß-pinene), citrus (d-limonene), lavender (linalyl acetate), rosemary

(8-cineole), peppermint (carvones), rose petals (rose oxide), cedar, cypress and juniper (cedrol).[13]

So, what happens when we sniff these different plant scents? Which specific mechanisms and pathways are triggered in our bodies, and what cocktail of smells emitted by plants have strong scientific evidence to show that, when we do so, it leads to improved health outcomes?

I was surprised to discover that there are still relatively few plant groups for which the effect of smelling specific plant volatile organic compounds have been properly scientifically determined.[14] In the following section I summarise some of this ongoing research, focusing on scents which we commonly encounter in our everyday lives, including various conifers, citrus fruits, herbs (lavender, rosemary, mint) and roses. These four groups appear to have some of the strongest scientific evidence and/or results indicating potentially important health outcomes when we smell them. I suspect that by the end of this chapter, you will never smell certain plants in the same way again – and you might well be heading out to buy a room diffuser and scented plant oils, or even find yourself chopping up lemons more regularly.

Conifers

Conifers give us some of the most recognisable and evocative scents in the plant kingdom, from a walk in a shady pine forest to the fragrant Christmas tree. In fact, they are also some of our most ancient trees.

Conifer trees first appeared in the fossil record around 310 million years ago, with eight different conifer families still existing today.[15] Conifers are an extraordinarily diverse group of trees with species growing in different environments all over the world, and none more so than the Pinaceae, the largest conifer family with around 232 different species and the most widespread globally. Pinaceae trees are found on almost every continent of the world except Antarctica – although interestingly, they had a dominant presence on that continent too when it was ice-free around sixty million years ago.[16] Well-known tree species in this family include fir (*Abies*), spruce (*Picea*), pine (*Pinus*) and larch (*Larix*).

There are a number of features used to distinguish the Pinaceae family, including simple needle-like leaves, but the one most relevant here is that many of them release a scent made up of a distinctive set of aromatic monoterpenes; the pinenes (α-pinene and ß-pinene) and limonene (d-limonene). It is these monoterpenes in the air that create the unmistakable smell we encounter when walking through a conifer forest, or even in pine furniture. Like other natural scents, its smell is often used to add an attractive pungency to household products such as soaps and bathroom cleaner.

In the natural environment, pinene is released in such vast quantities that you might even see it, because it reacts with sunlight and ozone to form the characteristic haze sometimes apparent above pine and spruce forests in the sun.

Hints that smelling these compounds could have important effects on our physiological and psychological well-being first emerged in studies associated with the practice of forest bathing in the 1990s.[17] Here, experiments showed that spending time in coniferous forests was associated with a whole raft of health benefits including improved cardiovascular function, enhanced immunity, reduced inflammatory indices and better emotional state and attitude.[18] However, as is the case with a lot of the forest bathing experimentation, it was difficult to separate the role that smell played in these outcomes from other aspects of the forest environment such as shape of vegetation, colour and sound.

To address this issue, a series of experiments was established in clinical settings, first by the same scientists carrying out the forest bathing experiments, and then in other laboratories across South-east Asia, the US and the UK.[19] The huge advantage of using these clinical settings is that other factors (sight, sound and so on) can be controlled.

One of the most simple of these studies was carried out by Professor Harumi Ikei and colleagues from the University of Chiba in 2016.[20] They set up an experiment where ß-pinene and α-pinene was dispersed from a funnel near participants' noses for ninety seconds, and a suite of physiological and psychological parameters were measured while this was happening. The same experiment was then run again, but this time using air without this compound in it. The order of smelling the air/scent was also switched so that some participants smelt it first, followed by the non-scented air, while for others it was the other way round. The impact on the participants' nervous system was assessed via heart-rate variability, and the volunteers were asked to subjectively evaluate how the two smells affected their mood and levels of anxiety.

What emerged were strongly significant results even after only ninety seconds of smelling air infused with α-pinene, showing an increase in parasympathetic heart-rate variability (which is known to increase during relaxation) and a reduction in the rates of heartbeat. Both measurements indicate that smelling air infused with α-pinene can quickly induce physiological relaxation. The participants also reported that they felt more comfortable and less anxious after smelling the air infused with α-pinene.

While these experiments in laboratory settings are interesting and important, the practical question arises of whether we also get benefits when we are outside, breathing these compounds at levels that are found in the ambient air, for example when walking in a forest? Also, does more equal better? If the concentration of the compounds increases, do the health benefits associated with it also increase? This latter point is, I think, particularly interesting, because different combinations of trees in a forest and seasonal variations in air temperature mean that we are often walking through a constantly changing smell landscape. Next time you are walking in a forest, stop and smell the air in different locations, and you will see (or smell) what I mean. There are subtle differences even within a single forest. Understanding the smellscape is important if we are serious about designing forests for health and well-being.

I was therefore delighted to come across an experiment carried out in 2019 by researchers from Konuk University in South Korea.[21] They examined the response of participants to smelling air infused with different concentrations of the monoterpenes α-pinene, ß-pinene and d-limonene at levels that are naturally found in forest ambient air. They chose four increasing levels of concentrations of odour that we detect as a 'pine-like' smell when we encounter it in a room or in a forest. The effect of the scents on the

Pinene and limonene on brainwave activity and heart-rate variability

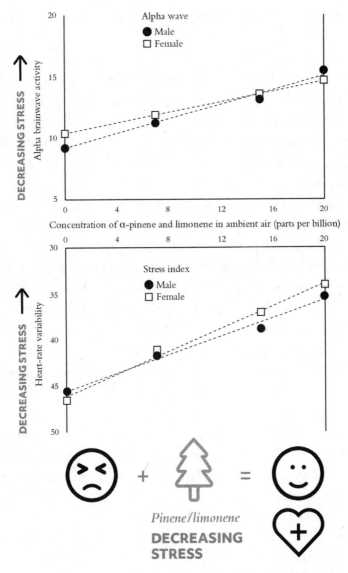

Source: H. Ikei, C. Song and Y. Miyazaki.

97

participants' brain-wave activity and heart-rate variability were measured, along with a questionnaire to self-evaluate mood.

Fascinating results emerged. There was a strong positive linear relationship between alpha brain-wave activity and concentrations of the volatile organic compounds in the air, meaning that as the concentrations in the air increased, the participants' alpha brain wave became more enhanced, indicative of an increasingly relaxed state. Similarly, there was a strongly negative linear relationship between stress levels detected in heart-rate variability and concentrations of α-pinene, ß-pinene and d-limonene. So, the more scent in the air, the less stress encountered − at least up to the levels measured in this experiment. Higher concentrations of these compounds in the air also appeared to indicate improved psychological well-being: whereas 44 per cent of the participants said that they felt comfortable when there was the minimum concentration in the air, this increased to 93 per cent when the concentrations increased to levels where the air had a detectably strong pine-like smell in it.

This last aspect of the experiment, and similar findings from others, are not however without their critics. Some have argued that these psychological reactions could be more to do with the influence of previous experiences, assumptions and prejudices associated with the odour. How do we know that people feeling more relaxed when smelling certain scents is not caused by simply associating the smell with previous pleasant experiences?

To tackle this question requires testing the smell on participants with no previous experience of it. Difficult to do, one might think − until two scientists came up with the ingenious idea of seeing what happens when we try these smells out on babies.[22] Seventeen infants aged between one and three and a half months old were 'volunteered' by their mothers for this experiment and exposed to two minutes each of air infused with three different aromas. The first contained odours of α-pinene, the second d-limonene and the third had no aroma and therefore acted as a control. While inhaling these different airs, the babies' heartbeat rate was recorded as a basic measure of level of stress. And the findings were clear. When smelling the odour of d-limonene, there was a clear decrease in the infants' heartbeat rate, taken to indicate that they became more relaxed.[23] In contrast, there was no such response to the control (no smell) or, curiously, when smelling α-pinene. The response to d-limonene therefore suggests that this reaction is indeed innate and independent of any influences from previous experience. Why there was a lack of response with α-pinene remains unclear. One suggestion is that this could be because the olfactory system is relatively undeveloped in infants, and that some smells might not therefore have the same impact as in adults. This is something that certainly warrants further investigation.

The take-home message from these various studies is that we should all be seeking out pine forests for our recreational walks (or sniffing pine-scented oils and soaps) – and the more conifers, the better. It will make us calmer and more relaxed. There does indeed appear to be a scientifically measurable response involved in our instinctive feelings of relaxation and reduced stress.

While making us more relaxed is important for our physical and mental health, there is another and potentially far more important change that occurs when we smell the scent from another family of conifers: the Cupressaceae family, in particular cypress and juniper.

The woody/peppery smells released by trees such as cypress and juniper are created by very large terpenoid molecules called sesquiterpenoids. These have fifteen carbon atoms in their structure, which means that they are slower to release their smell as a gas into the air but are also more persistent in our noses when we smell them. Cypress and juniper have a smell that is composed predominantly of a suite of sesquiterpenoids called ß-cadinene and cedrol, along with concentrations of the monoterpenes α-pinene, ß-pinene and d-limonene.

A number of important clinical experiments now demonstrate that inhaling these compounds can trigger involuntary neural responses that result in significant reductions in heart rate and in levels of stress hormones in saliva and brain activity, indicating physiological relaxation.[24] This is important in itself. However, there is another feature of smelling the scent from these trees that I find particularly remarkable: its apparent ability to increase levels of natural killer cells in our blood. Killer cells play a major role in the host-rejection of virally infected cells and cancer tumours. Clearly a simple, natural way of getting more of them has to be worth investigating.

Natural killer cells are a type of cell called a lymphocyte. They directly seek out and kill certain kinds of malignant cells including those causing tumours and cells infected with viruses. They do this by producing anti-cancer proteins, such as perforin and granzyme. These proteins then kill the target tumour/virus-infected cells by triggering

BEFORE and AFTER measurements of adrenaline hormone and natural killer cells

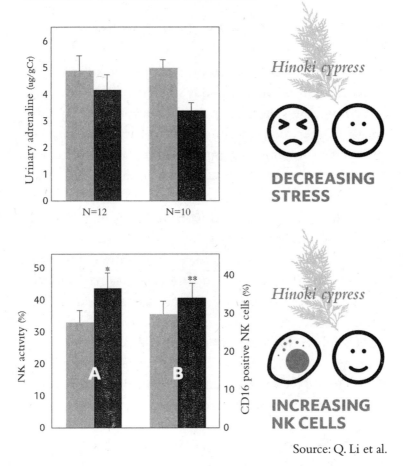

Source: Q. Li et al.

apoptosis, a naturally occurring process involving a series of molecular steps that leads to the death of these cells.

An extraordinary study carried out by Quin Li and colleagues from the Nippon Medical School in Tokyo showed that when participants spent three consecutive nights in a hotel room that had the scent of Japanese Hinoki cypress (*Chamaecyparis obtusa*) diffused in the air, not only was there a significant reduction in adrenaline hormone in their urine, but there was also a significant increase of natural killer cells in their blood.[25]

Given the central importance of natural killer cells to human health and our own body's system of fighting cancers and viruses, I was therefore somewhat surprised to find that, ten years after this experiment, there have been relatively few others following up on the potential of plant scents in this respect. Perhaps this research has been missed, or there is still a certain reluctance among medical scientists in the era of all things genomic to work on what might be seen as 'basic' plant compounds. I don't know. But, interestingly, further research is starting to emerge around this topic, including a study published in 2018 in *Oncotarget* – a journal specifically focused on oncology and cancer research.[26] The findings should make all of us head for cypress forests – or at least diffuse this scent in our rooms at home.

Professor Tsung-Ming Tsao and colleagues from the Experimental Research Forest of National Taiwan University looked at health benefits associated with inhalation of the scent from Japanese cedar (*Cryptomeria japonica*). They looked at two types of interaction with the smell: first, the impact of everyday inhalation resulting from living near forests containing these species; and second, what happens when we take a walk in a cypress forest. They first examined the concentration of natural killer cells in the blood of 90 university colleagues who lived in houses situated in a forested environment and compared their bloods with 110 colleagues who lived in an urban environment not near to a forest. They then examined the bloods and cardiovascular health of 25 individuals who went on a five-day/four-night trip in Xitou Experimental Forest in Taiwan. This forest contains many Japanese cypress trees, and as a result has high levels of the volatile organic compound cedrol in the ambient air.

Both sets of data from the participants' bloods yielded strongly significant findings. First, the percentage of natural killer cells was significantly higher in the group that lived near the forest than in the urban group, and in particular in overweight men with hyperglycaemia. From this, the authors drew the preliminary conclusion that the immune response of people with specific cardiovascular risk factors may be improved by living in homes close to a forest environment emitting these volatile organic compounds. Second, and possibly even more significant, was the finding that those who went on the trip to the forest for five nights had a significant increase in natural killer cell activation. And importantly, these elevated levels of natural killer cells in their blood lasted for more than seven days after the trip ended.

These findings, and several others, clearly indicate that inhaling Cupressaceae scent can enhance our immune system, in this case by elevating the number of natural killer cells.[27] Importantly, these effects are not just immediate but have a legacy effect that can last days, and may even confer health benefits over periods measurable in years.

Citrus

A second group of volatile organic compounds that now have strong evidence for health benefits when we smell them are those emitted by citrus fruits: oranges, lemons, limes, grapefruits, mandarins and tangerines.

Fossil evidence suggests that plants in the citrus family (Rutaceae) first evolved more than eight million years ago in a triangle defined by modern-day north-eastern India, northern Myanmar and north-western Yunnan, in China. Over the next four million years, rapid radiation and diversification of citrus occurred, resulting in species such as citron, pomelos, mandarins, kumquats and papedas appearing across the south and south-east Asian peninsula, the Tibetan Plateau, Japan and Australia.[28]

Somewhat later, around the third century BCE, citrus species spread west into Mediterranean Europe via various trading routes. By this time, citrus fruit was recognised as an important economic commodity and one that represented high social status if you were able to acquire it. For example, excavated fossil seeds and other remains of lemon (*Citrus limon*), dating to the late first century BCE or early first century CE, have been found in the gardens of high-ranking members of the Roman Empire. And it was not just early European populations that saw the economic potential of these plants; archaeological evidence indicates that citrus species were being cultivated and eaten in India and in China as early as the Xia dynasty (2100–1600 BCE). Citrus species were also a prized commodity for use in essential oils, spices, preservatives and perfumes, demonstrating that smell was highly valued alongside applications such as cookery and ornamental gardens.

Among the characteristic features of citrus plants in the Rutaceae family, two stand out: their distinctive fruit and their smell.[29] First, the fleshy fruit of citrus is quite unlike any other family. It consists of a leathery outer part covered with oil glands, a spongy thick middle part (this is the white pithy part of an orange or lemon) and an inner membrane with juicy, thin-stalked pulp vesicles. What is probably less well known is that the pulpy bits in an orange, within which the seeds are embedded, are in fact modified hairs. I will never look at the insides of an orange or lemon in the same way again. Second, their characteristic scent is due to translucent glands and cells that contain volatile oils in many parts of the plant, particularly in the skin of the fruit.

The distinctive smell comes from a volatile organic compound called d-limonene. As mentioned above, d-limonene is also released in the scent of some conifers; but occurs in its most highly concentrated form in the skin of citrus fruits. And, like other terpenes, manufactured versions of d-limonene are used extensively in everyday products from food flavourings and perfumes to soaps, hand cleansers, shower gels and shampoos.

As with conifers, as well as leading to a reduction in stress, smelling d-limonene can also alter the biochemical pathways that inhibit the effect of inflammatory cells and other inflammation pathways in the lungs. This type of inflammation is characteristic of that associated asthma, bronchitis and chronic obstructive pulmonary disease. The scent of lemon peel in easing these symptoms of asthma and other illnesses is therefore of great interest.[30] Interestingly, preliminary studies have also indicated that d-limonene can be conveniently given as an inhalation since it is easily absorbed and used by the body, and therefore can potentially provide direct and quick reduction of inflammation in the respiratory tract.[31]

Even though the majority of the work to date has been carried out on mice rather than humans, the significance of the health benefits associated with smelling d-limonene are clear. I am no medic, but I do wonder if in years to come, smelling or inhaling the scent from lemons and other citrus fruits might become one option for treating mild respiratory tract inflammation. This is already being suggested by some researchers.[32]

Herbs (lavender, rosemary and mint)

A third group of scent compounds with clearly indicated health benefits have provided the subject matter for folksongs, nursery rhymes, the cries of street vendors and the lyrics of poets since time immemorial: sweet-smelling herbs, including lavender, rosemary and mint.

These species are all found in the plant family Lamiaceae, known for its deeply aromatic scented leaves, which are usually leathery to touch and sometimes have serrated edges, making them look a bit like nettles (although nettles specifically are in a different plant family called Urticaceae). The earliest fossil records date evolution of Lamiaceae family to around 100 million years ago, probably originating in South-east Asia.

Lavender is associated with relaxation and sleep. There are around forty-seven different species of lavender in the Lamiaceae family, found all over the world. To us, the word usually conjures up the distinctive scent of the common lavender, sometimes known as English lavender (*Lavandula angustifolia*). This smell is created by a group of volatile organic compounds called terpenoid esters, including the compounds linalyl acetate and linalool. It is the combination of these two compounds that is responsible for the distinctive woody aroma of lavender.[33]

Lavender has long been used in aromatherapy and massage oils to enhance relaxation. It is now also commonly sold as an essential oil or in a spray to use on pillows to aid sleep. But, as one recent scientific publication noted rather sniffily, these types of therapies and interventions are not always accepted by mainstream scientists.[34]

Are they right? Is this just pseudoscience, or does it have any basis in evidence? When researching this question, I not only came away reassured that money spent on lavender spray for insomnia is a good investment, but also that we should all have lavender puffing out from diffusers in our offices to ward off the impact of stress.

Dealing with anxiety first, over the past decade there have been a number of experiments showing the efficacy of lavender for alleviating stress in real-life situations.[35] These have included, for example, trials looking at the responses of patients with ongoing pain or before undergoing a range of medical procedures, from people undergoing chemotherapy and open-heart surgery to women with painful pre-menstrual symptoms. Researchers put the data from twenty-four trials together, so that the results could be quantitively compared. They found strong and convincing clinical evidence that when we inhale lavender scents, it triggers changes in our nervous and endocrine systems and mental state, leading to physiological and psychological calming.[36]

As well as enhancing emotions and feelings, when we smell lavender scents, the volatile organic compound linalool passes into our blood. Scientific evidence indicates that this can then influence biochemical pathways in a similar way to when taking anxiolytic and sedative drugs such as benzodiazepines.[37] Although to date this has only been demonstrated in mice, it hints that lavender scent can help anxiety reduction. Such a natural approach will also certainly be a considerably cheaper alternative to prescription drugs.

I was also curious to know whether, as well as helping us to nod off, lavender can affect the quality of our sleep? This is important to understand because poor quality of sleep, with many wakeful episodes and 'light' periods of sleep, is related to a whole raft of health issues and even a shorter lifespan.

So, what is the effect of lavender on our sleep quality? A particularly nice study was carried out in 2021 by a team from the Faculty of Medicine in National Yang-Ming University in Taipei.[38] In this they measured the brain-wave activity of healthy participants while they slept for two nights. On one of these nights the aroma of lavender was released into the air. On the other, the control, there was no aroma. The participants were unaware of which night the aroma had been released.

What they found was a clear difference between the night when they were exposed to lavender scent compared to the control night. When sleeping with the lavender aroma in the air, the participants had long intervals of enhanced delta power in their brain-wave activity and reduced intervals of alpha power. This is important because delta power brain-wave activity in sleep EEGs is sometime referred to as slow-wave sleep and indicates good sleep quality. In comparison, alpha power usually indicates sleep interruptions and poor sleep quality. Lavender aroma leads to longer intervals of better-quality sleep.

These studies and many similar ones are now providing the sort of scientific evidence needed to change the conversation around lavender. It is not pseudoscience to suggest that its smell can make us calmer. Quite the opposite. They provide exactly the sort of quantitative evidence of real practical benefit to anyone suffering from poor sleeping patterns – lavender aroma on our pillows can improve poor sleep quality and insomnia.

Another well-known species in the Lamiaceae family, rosemary (*Salvia rosmarinus*), has the opposite effect: it helps keep us awake and alert. This is just as important for our health, well-being and productivity.[39]

Rosemary is native to the Mediterranean. Its distinctive smell is due to a predominance of a terpene called 1-8-cineole, along with pinene and camphor.[40] Why and how smelling rosemary scent keeps us awake is still under investigation, but a line of research that is yielding some interesting results shows that it may be due to the influence of these compounds on other biochemical pathways in our blood. Preliminary clinical experiments have shown that when we have elevated levels of 1-8-cineole compounds in our blood (i.e. from rosemary scent inhalation) they can inhibit the action of two enzymes that normally break down neurotransmitters in the brain responsible for alertness and arousal and are also implicated in conditions such as dementia.[41] By inhibiting these enzymes, the life of these neurotransmitters in our brain is therefore prolonged, meaning that we stay awake and alert for longer.

Can something as simple as rosemary scent therefore be used in everyday situations to keep us awake and more cognitively alert? A neat practical test was carried out in 2021 by researchers in the Birjand University of Medical Sciences in Iran to answer this question. They placed a few drops of rosemary scent inside facemasks worn by nurses on a night shift. A control group wore facemasks that had drops of water in them.[42] Eighty shift-working nurses took part, and completed questionnaires specifically designed to test sleepiness and alertness before and after the night shift. Clear results emerged showing that the participants who inhaled the rosemary scent reported greater alertness and decreased sleepiness.[43] This is something we could all easily try out in our own daily lives, particularly in situations requiring long periods of concentration.

Last in this fragrant group of plants in the Lamiaceae family which show evidence of clear benefits when we smell them, are the mints, including spearmint (*Mentha spicata*), peppermint (*Mentha piperita*) and pennyroyal mint (*Mentha pulegium*). The compounds responsible for the familiar minty aroma are a cluster of volatile organic compounds called the carvones. And there is increasingly strong scientific evidence that inhalation of peppermint can significantly improve both our alertness and our memory. A particularly nice study demonstrating this was one where some participants wore a peppermint-infused skin patch for six hours while undertaking a series of memory tests. A control group wore a blank patch. Those wearing the mint patch did much better.[44] Self-assessment questionnaires also used in this study indicated that the peppermint patch participants felt more alert compared to those wearing the blank patch. Many people already find that sucking peppermints and/or chewing peppermint gum helps them concentrate: maybe it's as much the smell as the action which has this effect.

Roses

Finally, any research into the effects of plant scents would not be complete without mention of roses. I love the smell of roses, and people-watching in the park suggests that many share my enthusiasm. It was therefore very satisfying to discover that these wonderful scents can also do us good.

The Rosaceae family contains a large number of well-known other genera including *Prunus* (peaches, plums, cherries, almonds and so on) and *Malus* (apples, pears, quinces and so on). It is the genus *Rosa* from which all our ornamental varieties of rose descended. Fossil evidence suggests that roses originated in central Asia and were first cultivated in gardens in China from around 5,000 years ago and then in modern-day Syria and Iran from around 3,000 years ago. Their popularity spread into the Roman Empire with evidence that the Romans used them for multiple purposes, including as confetti at celebrations, for ingredients in cooking, as medicines and in perfume. In the following centuries multiple blooming cultivated roses arrived in Europe along the trade routes from China. Nowadays there are known to be around 250 different species of roses globally and around 18,000 hybrid cultivars.

One surprising fact I came across, however, is that of all the rose species currently documented, only ten to fifteen species have contributed to the modern versions we have in our gardens and less than 10 per cent are known to have a clearly discernible scent.[45] Scented varieties include well-known garden roses such as Chinensis, Climber, English rose, Floribunda, Hybrid Tea, Multiflora, Damask, Musk rose, Polyantha, Rugosa and Shrub. And their wonderful smells are a result of them emitting over 400 volatile organic compounds with different concentrations and combinations resulting in the subtle differences between species. These compounds contain terpenes including citronellol, geraniol, eugenol and linalool.[46] However, the distinctive rose scent that they all have is actually from a different group of volatile organic compounds called the phenylpropanoids.[47]

So, what effect does smelling a rose have on us? Given the importance of roses to us as a garden flower, as cut flowers in our home and sometimes as a symbol of love, there is in fact remarkably little research looking into our responses when we smell these lovely blooms. However, one experiment carried out a few years ago confirmed what many of us would have suspected: smelling the scent of fresh roses, even for just ninety seconds, has a positive impact on physiological and psychological indicators of stress in our bodies.[48]

But can smelling roses also be used in a practical way? There is one study that has looked at this and has to be one of my favourite studies on the effects of smell, with clear and easily achievable potential benefits for a common activity: driving. This study looked at the effect of different smells on our driving behaviour, specifically at whether there were any differences apparent in our driving behaviours if we smelt the aromas of roses, peppermint, civet and, as a control, fresh air, while behind the wheel.[49]

In this study, designed by researchers in the department of Engineering and Informatics at the University of Sussex, participants were tested in a simulated driving environment, not on actual roads (thank goodness), and were assessed for their performance in elements like speeding and lane movements, while being challenged with a series of anger-inducing road events (erratic pedestrian, zigzagging car, cyclists and other cars cutting across their path). Various psychological tests were performed before and after the time in the simulator to see if smelling these scents had any effect.

Fascinatingly, their findings showed that both roses and peppermint scent in cars has the potential to influence driving behaviours in a positive way. Rose was the best; when smelling this scent, drivers had the lowest average driving speed (among all conditions), no crashes, and reported that they felt more relaxed and cautious when driving. Hallelujah.

Smelling peppermint scent was also good, but not as good as roses. Results showed that participants maintained the same speed as the control and reported feeling more alert. This finding is in line with other studies showing that smelling peppermint while driving helps people focus on the task and can improve reaction times. However, the number of simulated crashes in this experiment was not significantly different compared to the control (no scent): a less good outcome than smelling rose scent.[50]

Another important finding, especially in terms of road rage management, was that both rose and peppermint scents had a calming effect while people were driving and could make angry drivers happier and less stressed. In contrast, and somewhat worryingly, smelling civet resulted in a significantly higher number of collisions, faster speeds and more lane deviations.

At the beginning of this chapter, I found myself following several famous sets of footsteps up the panelled staircase of the headquarters of Edward Bodenham's family firm, Floris perfumiers. All of my shadowy predecessors up those stairs had been looking for the same thing: benefits derived from using the scents and smells of nature in our everyday lives. This chapter has looked into the science behind that impulse. While Edward's customers thought they were simply buying a pleasing olfactory element to add to their daily lives, science has begun to look at whether our sense of smell can bring more substantial benefits to our health. Will the perfumiers' shops of the future be stocked with bottles whose labels list their effect in reducing stress and boosting killer-cells, and be staffed by sales assistants who are also medics?

I think it would be fair to say in conclusion that research into protective plant perfumes is still in its scientific infancy. Research into this important topic is only carried out by relatively few laboratories in the world, and large-scale clinical trials have yet to be instigated – although there is a noticeable increase in research papers on this topic over the past three to five years, so maybe these will now be forthcoming. Why research into the impact of different plant scents is so far behind that into other senses is a mystery to me; but clearly it is an area that has huge potential health benefits. Smelling the right plant scents can not only reduce anxiety and levels of stress, but also inflammatory responses, and enhance our immune systems through the elevation of natural killer cells in our blood. Even if the large clinical trials are still lacking, I personally think some of this evidence is strong enough to start including more of the scents in our everyday lives to gain the protective perfumes provided by nature.

But don't share your car with a civet cat.

5

Sound Surgery: From Birdsong to Rustling Leaves

Noise-cancelling headphones are one of my favourite modern inventions. They suppress unwelcome noise and boost music, or even just silence. The science behind them is relatively straightforward: they contain a small microphone that captures the background sound, and a small amplifier that generates sound waves that are exactly out of phase with this background noise. When the two sets of sound waves collide, they cancel each other out. Result: silence. Perfect. And simple.

But why do we need to shut out noise? And what is bad noise? Conversely, what is good noise, and how do we find it? Not for the first time in this book, the answer lies in nature.

Sadly, we don't all have the luxury of owning noise-cancelling headphones. But if the emerging evidence base on the impact of sounds on our health is correct, their selective approach to sound is something we all need. In particular, we now know that some sounds can have a strongly negative impact on our health. And it is not just auditory damage caused by an excessive volume of the sound. There is strong scientific evidence to indicate that regular exposure to certain types of everyday sounds such as traffic, phones and planes is associated with increased occurrences of cardiovascular diseases, sleep disturbances, cognitive impairment in children, psychological disorders and even obesity.[1] Bad sound is bad for you.

Knowledge of these detrimental effects has led to policies in many cities across the world that set thresholds for volume, duration and time of day.[2] Somewhat bizarrely, there are also examples of authorities using 'bad' sounds as a weapon. For example, the FBI played Christmas carols at an excruciating volume to try to drive David Koresh and his Branch Davidian sect out of their compound in Waco, Texas, in 1993, and the US military has used music to wear down prisoners of war to such an extent that one notorious detention centre on the Iraq–Syria border became known as 'the disco'.

Of course, not all sounds are detrimental, and many may well be good for us. For example, recordings of 'sounds of nature' have been marketed for a long time in many different mediums, from piped music in yoga classes, to whale-song and the whispering of waves, with the promise that they will help us relax and even sleep.

But what actually happens to us when we listen to them? Unlike research into sounds that have a negative impact on our health, I think it would be fair to say that scientific research into good sounds has been largely absent until recently. However, an expanding research agenda is now emerging on how natural sound affects us physiologically and psychologically. And intriguing findings are emerging, not least that, sometimes, hearing nature has more positive impacts on our health than seeing it. So, what should we listen to and why?

We probably don't usually think much about our ears. Yet they are a remarkable and complex feature that allows the conversion of sound waves in the air into electrical signals, which then trigger neural activity in our brains.

In simple terms, our ears are made up of three sections called the outer, middle and inner ear. After sound waves enter the outer part of the ear (the odd-shaped bit on the sides of our head), they move through the ear canal to the ear drum, causing it to vibrate. These vibrations then pass into the middle ear where three tiny bones amplify them, and they pass into the inner ear.

The inner ear consists of a small snail-shaped structure called the cochlea, and this is where the action happens. The cochlea is filled with fluid and when the vibrations pass into it, they cause ripples that push against a membrane lined with thousands of tiny sensory hair cells. The movement of these hairs opens tiny pores, which release electrochemically charged particles (ions) generating electrical signals. These electrical signals are then transmitted via the auditory nerve to various regions in the brain where they trigger neural activity that leads to motor (movement), physiological (such as an increase in heart rate) and/or psychological (such as feeling happy) changes in response to a particular sound.

It is the last part of this process that is particularly important here: which sounds trigger responses that have a positive impact on our health and well-being? This question of good and bad sounds really came home to me recently when I was in a hotel lobby in the city of Brussels. The designer of this hotel had clearly decided that a natural 'jungle theme' was the best option for this space, complete with sounds of squawking parrots, growling lions and other more generic jungle-type sounds. These noises were certainly a distraction – both in the lobby area and while waiting for a very slow elevator to arrive – but did they have a beneficial effect on me or was my increase in frustration at both the check-in and waiting for the lift somehow linked to these noises?

Some of the earliest work to look at beneficial soundscapes in cities focused on whether we perceive certain sounds as relaxing and restorative. Over 1,000 Swedish participants living in the city of Gothenburg, for example, were asked to select statements that most closely aligned to how different everyday sounds made them feel. In their responses, strong agreement emerged in their perceptions of what sounds made them feel 'good' or 'bad', with the following three statements gaining most votes: 'Birdsong in the area makes me feel calm'; 'Rustling trees make me feel calm'; and 'Noise from the city and traffic interferes with my experience of the area'.[3]

That might seem like a complicated way of stating the obvious. That was my first reaction. But then I came across a series of further studies that looked at whether we perceive some sounds of nature as more restorative than others. This is where it begins to get interesting. It appears that we do.

For example, in a neat experiment, clear preferences emerged when Polish participants listened for one minute each to one of the following sounds, divided into groups of natural and urban as follows:

Nature sounds – blackbird in a clearing, blackcap in the woods, corncrake at a pond, crows, deer in rut, forest noises (boar and birds), frogs at a pond, great reed warbler, howling wolves, larks and barred warbler, meadow in the spring (many bird species), night in the woods (eagle-owls and wind), nightingale, ravens, river, robin at a river, sea, seagulls on a windy day, summer night (crickets and birds), swarm of insects, thunderstorm and wren at a stream.

Urban sounds – airport (aeroplane landing), street (ambulance), old town (barrel organ), café, amusement park (carousel), church bells, concert (orchestra tuning and applause), construction site, firework display, highway, ice rink (people skating), lawnmower, parade (brass band), roadworks (pneumatic hammer), fire department (siren), street noise, underground (empty underground carriage), swimming pool, traffic jam (with car horns), train, video arcade and wind chimes.

When the participants were then asked to rank these sounds for their perceived ability to promote recovery and restoration from stress and mental fatigue, clear findings emerged. As expected, all participants found sounds from nature much more favourable than urban sounds.[4] However, there was also strong agreement in the ranking of the different types of natural sounds. Sounds that contained birdsong were in the top five, including the sounds of a robin at a river, a wren at a stream, a blackbird in a clearing and a blackcap in the woods. And this is a finding that has been replicated time and again from studies across the world: birdsong is perceived as having the best restorative properties, followed by water (streams in woods, waves at a beach) and wind in trees.[5]

Natural sounds on health and positive affective outcomes

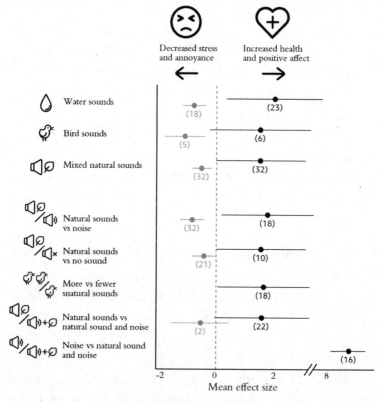

Source: R. T. Buxton, A. L. Pearson, C. Allou, K. Fristrup
and G. Wittemyer.

But is this the case for all bird species? Not necessarily. Eleanor Ratcliffe and colleagues from the University of Surrey played a variety of different bird sounds to volunteers. Perhaps unsurprisingly, they found that the cawing of crows and magpies was not perceived as restorative compared to a number of other species.[6] And it would appear that this

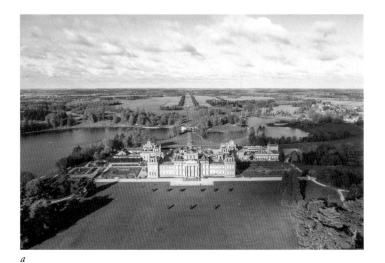

a

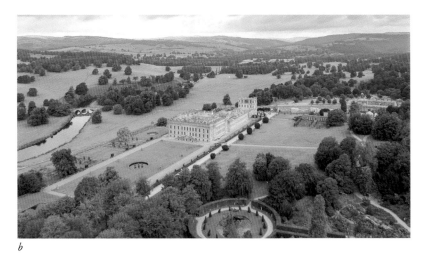

b

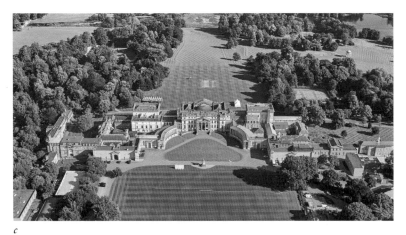

c

Three Capability Brown-designed gardens in England, see page 14: (a) Chatsworth House gardens in the Peak District; (b) Blenheim Palace gardens in Oxfordshire; (c) Stowe House gardens, Buckinghamshire.

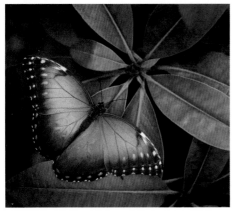

a

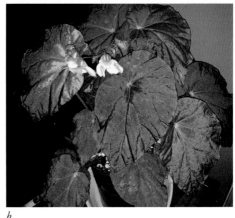

b

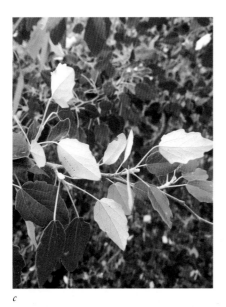

(a) The blue morpho butterfly (*Morpho peleides*) has micro-scales on its wings that selectively reflect blue light, leaving the other bandwidths to be transmitted through the wings, see page 46; (b) The irridescent sheen of a *Begonia pavonina* results from internal leaf microstructures, see page 46; (c) The top and bottom of white poplar leaves (*Populus alba*). The underside is covered in hairs which result in its white appearance, see page 46; (d) Varieties of English ivy (*Hedera helix*) with different coloured two-toned leaves. The differences in leaf colouration are due to genetic mutations, with each resultant variety having a very different colour combination, see page 53.

c

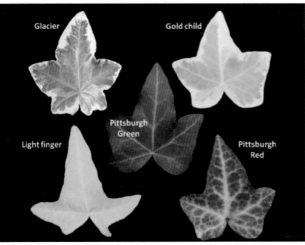

d

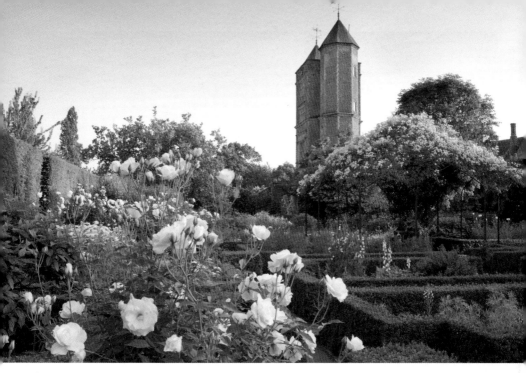

a

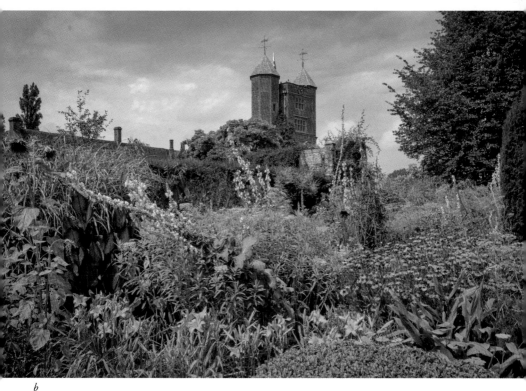

b

In Vita Sackville-West's gardens at Sissinghurst Castle in Kent, she used flower colours to design a number of small interconnective, yet distinctive, gardens, including for example the (a) 'white' garden, and (b) 'red' garden, see page 64.

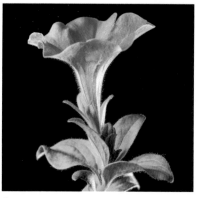

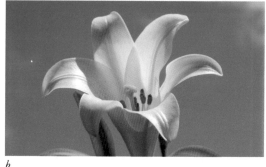

a

b

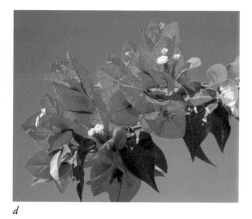

c

d

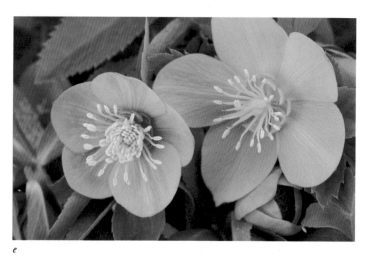

e

(a) The 'trumpet-like' shape of the petunia flower results from differential rates of cell division in the final stages of the petal's development, see page 68; (b) The characteristic curved petals of a lily flower stems from faster rates of cell division at the margins of the petal relative to those in the centre, resulting in a curved shape, see page 68; (c) The bright yellow in sunflowers (*Helianthus annus*) is due to the petals containing a carotenoid pigment called β-carotene, see page 70; (d) the red-purple varieties of bougainvillea flowers are due to betalain pigments, see page 70; (e) The presence of chlorophyll pigments in the petals of a green hellebore (*Helleborus viridis*) are responsible for its colour, see page 70.

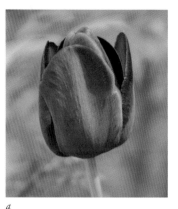
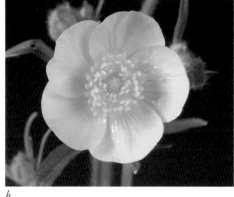

a

b

(a) The iridescent sheen of the 'Queen of the Night' tulip is caused by differential diffraction of light due to microstructural features on petal surface, see page 70; (b) Common buttercup, where the shiny appearance results from a double-mirror-like system, page 71; (c) Blue hydrangeas (*Hydrangea macrophylla*) grown in acidic soils; (d) Blue hydrangeas grown in alkaline soils, see page 70.

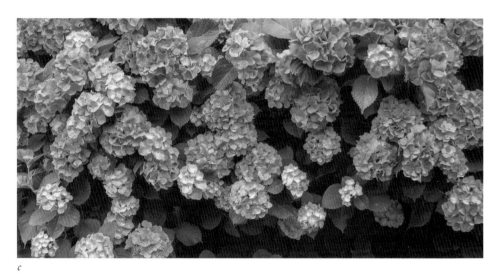

c

d

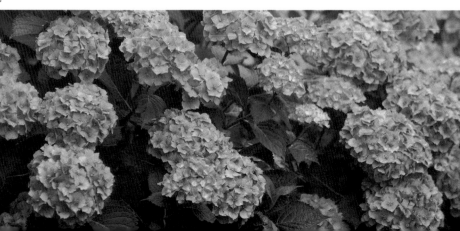

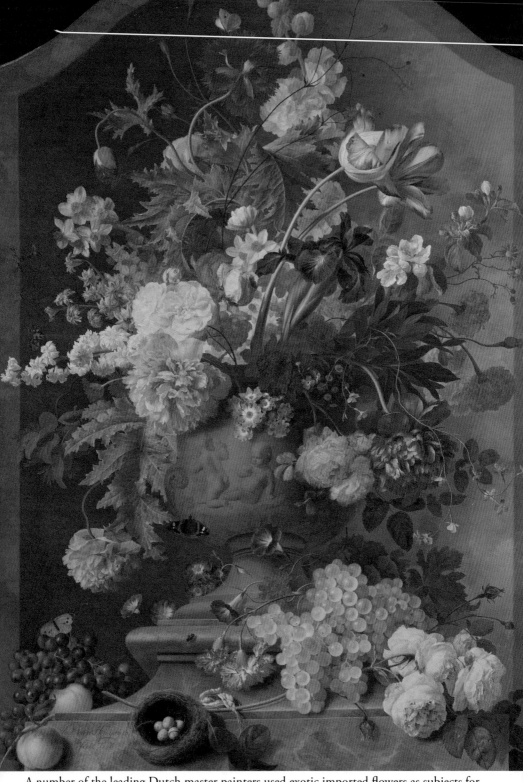

A number of the leading Dutch master painters used exotic imported flowers as subjects for their characteristic still-life paintings, including 'Flowers in a Terracotta Vase' painted by Jan van Huysum between 1736 and 1737, above, see page 72.

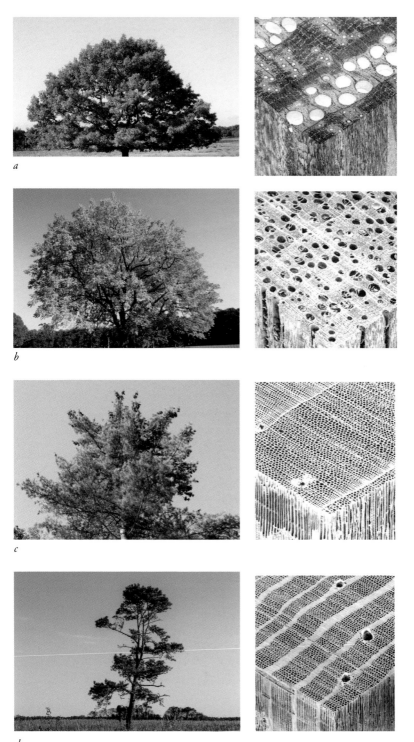

Showing common hardwood tree species (a) red oak (*Quercus rubra*) and (b) black walnut (*Juglans nigra*) and common softwood tree species; (c) Easter white pine (*Pinus strobus*); (d) southern yellow pine (*Pinus taeda*) and thin sections of their wood – note the difference in arrangement and size of pore structures in the wood, see page 147.

acetofi onde nelle febbri calide fi conuengono gli acetofi & i mezzani & non
dolci. Si chiamano aranci quafi aurantia poma che uuol dir pomi aurei o d'oro.

LIMONI.

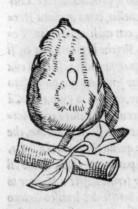

I LIMONI *nella facultà loro non fono molto di*
fcrepàti da i Cedri. Del fugo loro fe ne fa un firopo
utile a fpegner la caldezza della colera & nelle feb
bri contagiofe & peftilentiali. L'acqua fatta di limo
ni per lambico di uetro, oltr'all'adoperarfi dalle don
ne a pulirfene il uifo, guarifce le uolatiche, ouunque
elle fieno nella perfona & fimilmēte i pedicelli. Mef
fa ne gli firopi gioua mirabilmente alle febbri colle=
riche acute & contagiofe. Data a bere a fanciulli am
mazza i uermi del corpo, ilche fa anco il fugo fre=
fco, fpremuto dal frutto alla quantità d'una oncia piu
& māco fecōdo che fon grādi & piccioli i fanciullini.

LENTISCO.

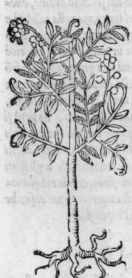

NASCE *il lentifco abondantemente in Italia, &*
fpecialmente nelle maremme di Siena, nafce nelle fu=
perbe, & antiche rouine Romane, & ueggonfene nel
la cofta di tutto il mare Tirrheno andādo uerfo Gae
ta, & uerfo Napoli infinitißime piante. Tra lequali
ue n'è affai di quello, che crefce, & s'ingroffa in arbo
ro, di quello, che fenza fare altro tronco, manda dalle
radici fpeßißimi farmenti, nel modo che fanno i nocci
uoli faluatichi. Ma è piu folto il lentifco ne rami, &
nelle frondi, & piu fi piega con le cime de farmenti
uerfo terra. Hanno l'uno & l'altro le frondi loro fi=
mili a quelle de i piftacchi, graffe, fragili, & uerdifcu
re, come che nelle eftremità loro, & in quella piccio=
la uena, che per lungo le fende, roffeggino affai. Il
lentifco è anchor egli di quelle piante, che non perdo
no mai le frondi, & però d'ogni tempo uerdeggia.
E la fua fcorza in tutta la pianta roßigna, uencida,
tenace, & arrendeuole. Produce oltre al frutto (come parimente fi uede nel tere=
binto) certi baccelli, come cornetti, piani, ne iquali è dentro un liquore limpido, il=
quale inuecchiandofi fi conuertifce in piccioli animaletti uolatili, fimili in tutto a
quelli che fi concreano nelle uefciche de gli olmi, & de terebinthi. Hanno le fron=

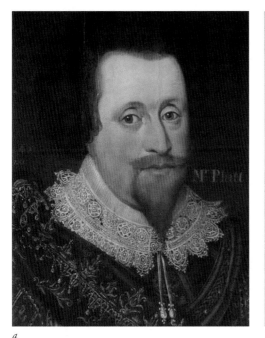

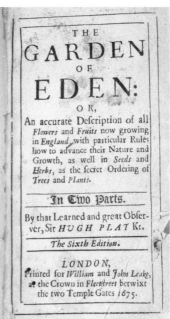

a   *b*

(a) Sir Hugh Plat (1552–1608) was widely attributed as having written the first domestic gardening handbook, *Floraes Paradise*, in 1608, which was reproduced for eighty years after his death under the title *The Garden of Eden*, see page 188; (b) Title page of *The Garden of Eden*; (c) A page from the book showing the detailed drawings and advice on cultivation of plants; (d) Anthurium (*Anthurium andreanum*) and (e) Peace Lily (*Spathiphyllum wallisii*) are examples of typical houseplants first imported from tropical regions in the mid-seventeenth century, see page 189.

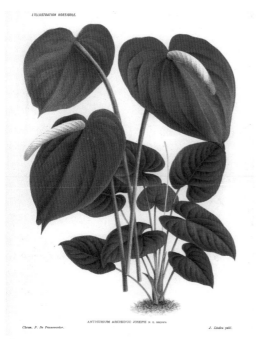

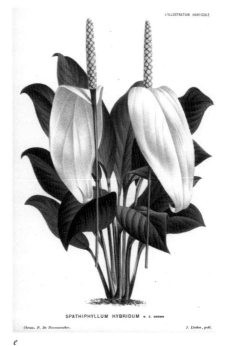

d   *e*

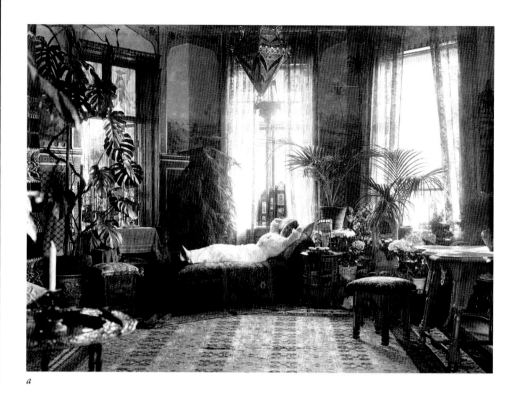

a

(a) Victorian sitting room complete with parlour palms, monstera plants and plant-inspired fabrics and furniture shapes; (b) Late 1950s sitting room with square-shaped furniture, checked curtains, and not a plant or plant-inspired fabric in sight, see page 190.

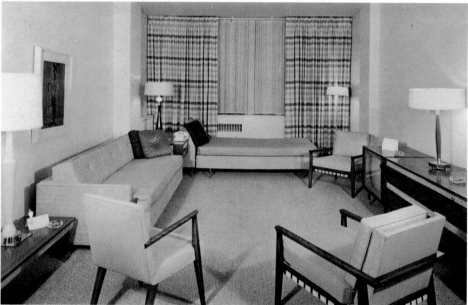

b

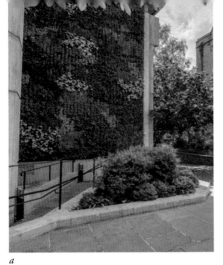

a

Green walls across the world from (a) St Edmund Hall at the University of Oxford to (b) Seoul's City Hall, with an indoor green wall so big it set a Guinness World Record as the world's largest vertical garden in 2013, see page 193; (c) Four different VR rooms designed to test the participants' physiological and psychological stress responses when spending time in them, see page 204.

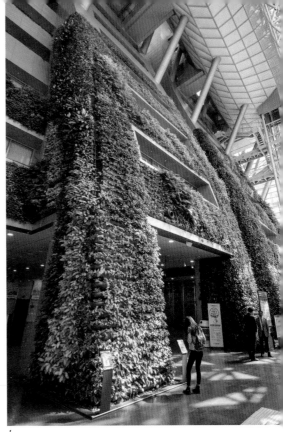

b

c

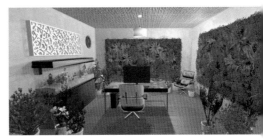

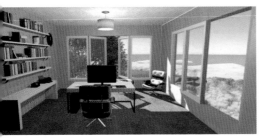

A: Non-biophilic

B: Indoor green

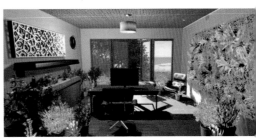

C: Outdoor view

D: Combination

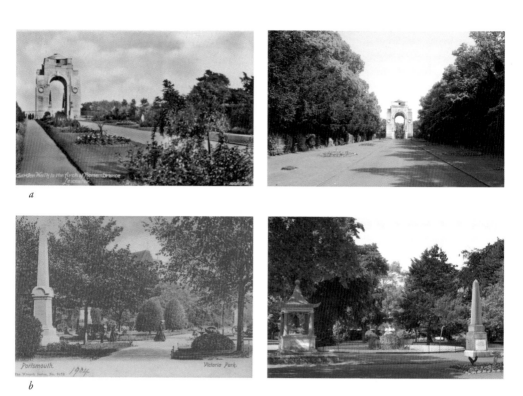

a

b

Victoria Parks in (a) Leicester and (b) Portsmouth. Both were planted in the late 1880s with formal herbaceous borders interspersed by lawns, and paths and ornamental features such as bandstands and drinking fountains. Many of these paths, features and structures are still in place in these parks today, see page 215.

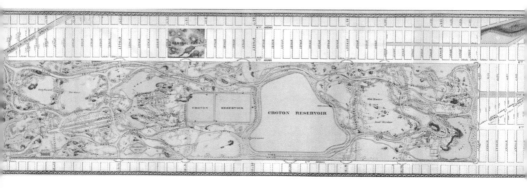

Original planting plans for New York's Central Park. Drawn in 1868 and opened in 1876 with a design focused on natural-looking planting and landforms including winding paths and lakes. Not a formal flowerbed in sight, see page 216.

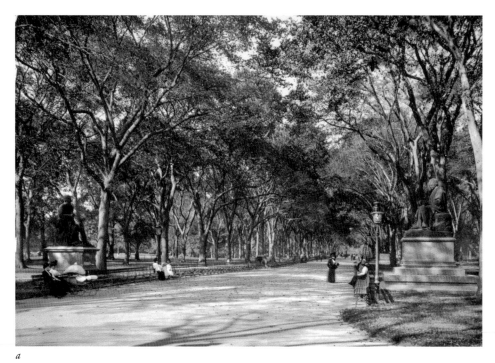

a

(a) The 'Mall' in Central Park in 1901; (b) The 'Mall' today, showing that this style of 'wilderness park' has been retained, see page 216.

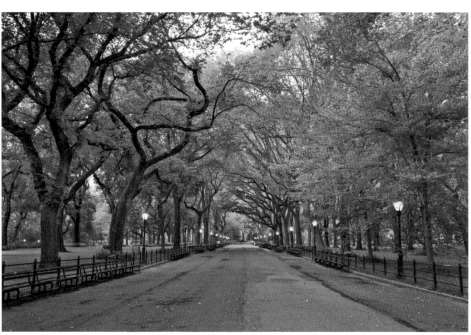

b

Common street trees and their distinctive leaves found in many cities across the world: (a) Maidenhair tree (*Ginkgo biloba*); (b) Plane trees (*Platanus* x *acerifolia*); (c) American sweet gum (*Liquidambar styraciflua*), see page 227.

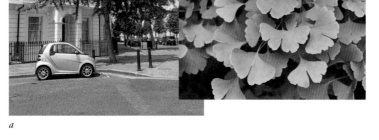

a

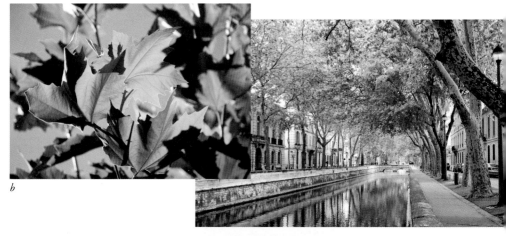

b

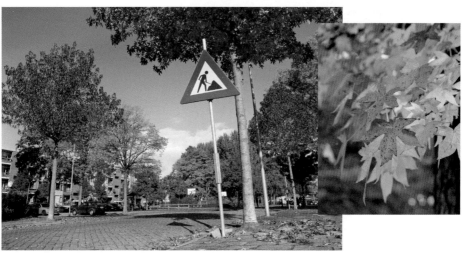

c

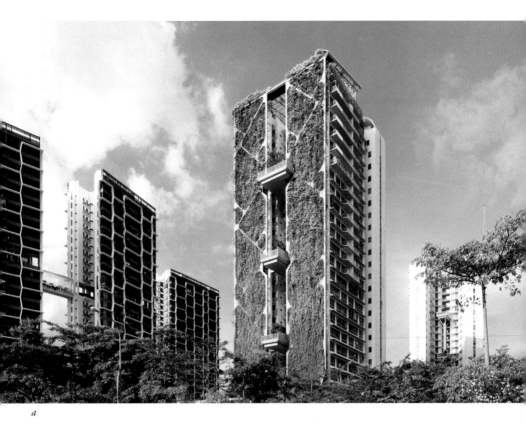

a

(a) CDL's Tree House in Singapore has the world's largest vertical garden (according to the Guinness World Records). The building's green wall measures ~24,640 square feet; (b) the world's tallest green wall is found growing 92m up the side of a residential building in Medellín, Colombia, see page 232.

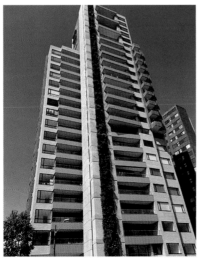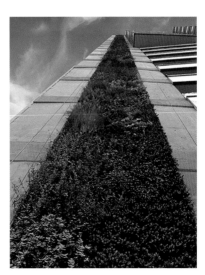

b

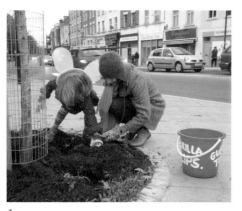
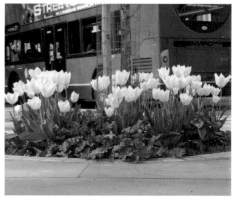

a

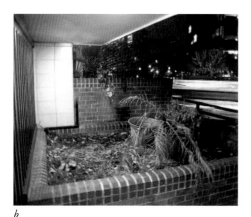
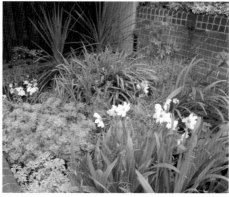

b

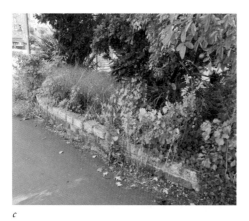
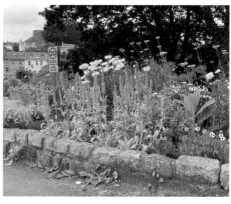

c

Gardening without boundaries: before-and-after photos of Richard Reynolds' guerrilla gardening projects in (a) Dulwich Road in Herne Hill, London; (b) Perronet House, Elephant and Castle, London; and (c) Station Road in Totnes, Devon, see page 246.

is not a culturally influenced preference; from the UK to Sweden and China, studies are showing that birds that have a loud screeching voice are unattractive to the human ear. In Sweden, for example, participants rated the distress call of lapwings or gulls or the cawing of black-headed gulls as not pleasant compared to the songs of birds such as chaffinches, and in China respondents to a questionnaire rated crows considerably less desirable and less restorative than woodpeckers and sparrows.[7] After my hotel lobby experience in Brussels, I would also place parrots in this category!

Why is this? What is it about some bird sounds that leads to these preferences? Is it something to do with the pitch, repeatability, volume or tone that is typically characteristic of different species?

One of my favourite technological innovations of recent years has been a series of smartphone apps that allow the user to identify wildlife from its calls and cries. You capture the background soundscape of birds, insects and animals through the microphone on your smartphone, and in return it tells you what species of frogs, crickets, bees, birds, bats and mosquitoes you are listening to. It's great fun, and hugely informative: I've learnt more about the wildlife I pass on my regular dog walks than I did from years of occasionally remembering to take a field guide or bird book with me.

My favourite is one developed by Cornell University that allows you to identify bird species from their song.[8] When you hear a bird singing you simply hold your phone up, press the record button, capture twenty seconds or so of the sound, press send, and within a minute or so, a message tells you what the bird is – a Shazam for birds. What the smartphone app is actually doing is capturing the acoustic wavelength of the song, its size, shape and pattern; its acoustic signature. This is then sent to a server where mathematical algorithms and machine learning compare the wavelength snippet to a library containing thousands of signatures of different bird species, along with other environmental information such as location and time of year, to enable the computer to identify the species and send the result back to the phone. It's an amazing feeling to think that you're drawing on this huge technological resource while standing in your local park wondering what that bird up in that tree is. And each use of the app adds another entry to the computer database, increasing the size and range of the electronic library against which other sounds can then be tested.

The system works because each bird species produces a distinctive acoustic signature. So, are there particular birdsong signatures that we find more restorative than others? This was the second question addressed by Ratcliffe and her colleagues.[9] They cleverly used data from a previous exercise where 174 participants had listened to and then ranked fifty different birdsongs from UK and Australian species for their perceived restoration potential.[10] Taking this ranked list, they analysed each of the birdsongs for their acoustic characteristics including harmonics, frequency, complexity of pattern and volume to see if certain songs that were ranked highly had distinctive acoustic patterns. Clear results emerged; birds that came the top of the list for perceived restoration potential, including blackbirds, dunnocks, blue tits, greenfinches and robins, had acoustic signatures that were tuneful but complex,

Seeing sound: acoustic signatures of different bird songs

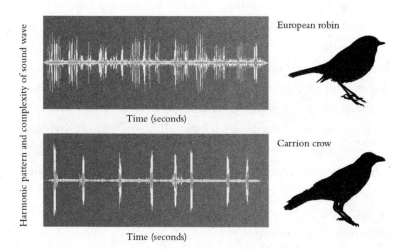

with repeated patterns at a comparatively low volume.[11] By contrast, those birdsongs ranked as being of lowest perceived restoration potential, including jays, herring gulls, silver gulls and kites, had little harmonic pattern or complexity and were much louder.

I don't think I will ever hear birdsong in the same way again. Yet one potential issue with these studies is that the majority are based on self-reported perception of the different birdsongs, usually obtained via questionnaires or other similar qualitative techniques. What I was therefore curious to understand further was how much of our perceived restoration potential of a sound translates into measurable changes in our bodies, for example in responses in our autonomic nervous system to stress or in our cognitive performance? Over the past decade a second tranche of clinically based studies have been looking at this question, showing that hearing certain sounds of nature can reduce physiological and psychological stress, improve our cognitive performance and even reduce levels of pain.

Looking at stress first, there are now a number of studies indicating that hearing certain natural sounds can bring about physiological calming.[12] For example, in one experiment, measurements of heart-rate variability and brain activity were taken of sixty-six participants who sat in a soundproof room and listened to five minutes each of four sounds: a forest with birds at dawn, waves on a beach on a calm sunny day, outdoor shopping streets with pedestrians and the cries of street vendors, and the noise of traffic at an intersection during peak rush-hour. Statistically strong differences emerged.[13]

Within one minute of hearing the birdsong and the ocean sounds, the participants became physiologically calmer. The longer they listened, the greater the reduction in markers of stress, at least for the full five minutes of the experiment. Hearing street and traffic sounds, meanwhile, increased levels of physiological stress. This suggests that the longer we listen, the more pronounced the effects, good and bad (though the effects over longer time periods of hours, or cumulative effects over months and years, have yet to be tested). This is clearly an important finding for safeguarding the health of people who work in noisy environments or live near busy roads.

Another finding to emerge recently is that hearing certain sounds of nature can also have a measurable impact on our cognitive performance. Plenty of people work with music in the background; but should we be listening to natural sounds instead? When undertaking tasks that require our directed attention, will we perform these quicker and more accurately if we listen to sounds of nature, as suggested by some?[14]

A study that beautifully demonstrates the potential cognitive benefits of listening to nature was carried out by Stephen Van Hedger and colleagues at the University of Chicago and published in a paper with the evocative title 'Of cricket chirps and car horns: the effect of nature sounds on our directed attention performance'.[15] In this experiment, they examined the difference in the cognitive abilities of participants after listening to twenty minutes of birdsong, moving water (rainfall, ocean waves), insects (cricket chirps) and wind, compared to listening to twenty minutes of traffic, café ambience with unintelligible speech and machinery (including the noise of an air-conditioning unit). Two tests were used to assess the participants' cognitive performance after hearing the nature and urban sound snippets. The first one involved working out orders of numbers backward (a so-called backward digit span test), the second, matching spoken letters and coloured boxes. In both cases, the speed taken to do the test and the number of mistakes made was used to assess the participants' levels of directed attention. Strong results emerged: when exposed to nature sounds, the tests were completed faster and with fewer mistakes.

The implications of this for the workplace or schools cannot be over-estimated, and should be an important area for future research.

A third important area where the science is offering up some very interesting results is the effect of hearing sounds of nature on our levels of pain. Pain is classically defined as an unpleasant sensory or emotional experience associated with actual or potential tissue damage. It is therefore both as a result of sensory triggers and of cognitive processing. In other words, it involves both real physical causes and our neurological and psychological response to those causes, at the same time.

Any surgery is stressful. Probably none more so than when we remain 'awake' under local or epidural anaesthetic. Even though it is clinically less risky, many studies have shown that the stress is considerable and can last for quite some time after the operation, and even prolong recovery rates. Finding natural ways to reduce stress caused during wakeful surgery has therefore been an area of research for a number of years. Early studies exploring the effect of playing music showed encouraging results: patients who listened to music during surgery felt less anxious. On a more parochial level, it's interesting to note that many high-street dentists appear to have known this for years and play soothing music in the surgery to relax and reassure nervous patients; doctors tend not to do this. However, these findings were often obtained anecdotally and did not provide the clear scientific evidence-base needed to make clinical decisions. Recently this has changed with a number of clinical studies now showing that, as well as music, sounds of nature might well provide important pain relief.

First was a study carried out in 2008 by a team of medical scientists from Toki General Hospital in Japan.[16] In this, patients who were undergoing a hernia repair under epidural anaesthesia were randomly assigned into one of two groups. The first group listened to a recording of leaves rustling in the wind and birds singing in springtime during their procedure. The second group listened to no sound, but the headsets chosen for this experiment were non-occlusive, meaning that the patients could hear and communicate with the anaesthesiologist and surgeon, so there was still background noise. To detect levels of stress, an enzyme in the patients' saliva called salivary amylase was measured. This is known to become raised in our saliva in response to physical as well as psychological stressors and is therefore often used as a clinical measure to determine stress levels. In this experiment salivary amylase activity was measured on arrival at the operating room and then again at the point of wound closure at the end of the operation.

Clear findings emerged: those patients who listened to the sounds of nature had significantly decreased salivary amylase activity at wound closure in comparison to those who heard no sound, indicating lower levels of stress.

The second experiment was carried out by a team of medical scientists on patients in hospitals in Iran.[17] They examined the influence of playing sounds of nature on headphones to people in hospital undergoing mechanical ventilation. Sixty patients in the intensive care unit of a teaching hospital in Tehran listened to ninety minutes of either the sounds of nature, or, as a control, silence. No sedation or painkillers were administered during the trial. Patients used a scale of 0–10 to score their pain, with no pain marked as 0 and highest pain level at 10, at intervals of thirty, sixty and ninety minutes. The results were clear. While all patients had a similar level of self-reported pain at the baseline, for each sequential timepoint, pain scores of those listening to sounds of nature fell and were significantly lower than in the control group. Even though the changes in pain scores were small, they were of clinical significance,

Mean pain over time

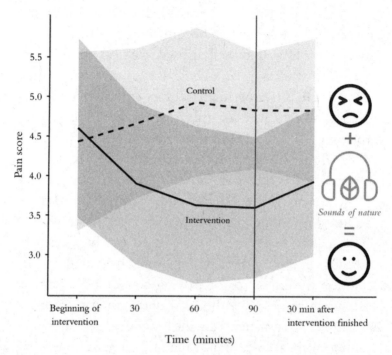

Source: V. Saadatmand et al.

and, as the authors concluded, indicate the large potential of listening to natural sounds to provide an easy, effective, safe, reliable and inexpensive way of reducing pain.

Similar findings were found in a third study carried out in a teaching hospital in Jahrom, Iran. Scientists examined the influence of natural sound on post-operative pain management in women who had undergone elective

Caesarean section.[18] Fifty-seven women took part over a ten-month period, with the experiment taking place eight hours after surgery (when most pain from the C-section surgery can occur). After their pain intensity was evaluated, using a similar scoring system to that described above, the women were divided into three intervention groups. One group were provided with headphones but no sound; the second group, headphones that played sounds of nature including birdsong, rain sounds, rivers, waterfalls and a walk through a jungle; and the third, no intervention at all. Pain assessments were undertaken at three intervals: twenty minutes into the intervention (while wearing headphones) and then fifteen and sixty minutes after the experiment (once headphones had been removed).

Again, clear results emerged. Those women who had listened to the nature-based sounds for twenty minutes had a significantly lower pain severity than the silent headphones and control group. Also, these reductions were more evident progressively fifteen and sixty minutes after the end of the intervention. Of note is the fact that those who wore headphones which produced no sound showed no difference in terms of perceived pain reduction from the women who had no intervention at all. This suggests that it was probably not the absence of unwelcome noise that was the deciding factor here, but the presence of natural sounds. This is clearly important for understanding the use of sound in pain management in an operative and post-operative environment.

All these studies indicate findings that are highly relevant to pain management. Nature-based sounds could play an important role in reducing post-operative pain by promoting physiological and psychological relaxation and diverting the patients' attention from anxiety, pain and negative experiences to more pleasant ones. This in turn will aid and facilitate recovery. This is clearly an area that warrants far greater attention and research.

Certain sounds of nature therefore appear to trigger pathways in our bodies that lead to significant improvements in cognitive abilities and reductions in levels of stress and even pain. But I was still a bit sceptical: are these just small, isolated examples? Or can they be translated into the bigger picture?

This concern was answered by an excellent synthesis of many studies looking at this question by Rachel Buxton and colleagues from Carlton University in Canada, published in the US journal *Proceedings of the National Academy of Sciences*.[19] In this horizon-scanning review they combined and reanalysed data from eighteen studies published in the past decade to see whether there was an overall link between hearing natural sounds and the rate and amount of improvement in physical and mental health and cognitive abilities. Between them, the studies reviewed involved many participants from eleven different countries, giving a large and varied dataset.

A staggering result emerged: listening to nature sounds resulted in improvements in health outcomes that were 1.8 times better (184 per cent) than those recorded in patients who heard urban sounds or no sounds at all. These improvements were apparent in both physiological and psychological measures including pain, heart rate, blood pressure, anxiety and depression.[20] They also found that, overall, there was a 28 per cent decrease in feelings of stress and annoyance in those exposed to natural sounds relative to the control groups. Another question Buxton and her colleagues asked in their analysis of this large dataset was whether certain types of natural sounds could be directly associated with specific benefits. They found that this was, indeed, the case. Intriguingly, water sounds had the largest effect in terms of improving our mood and cognitive performance, whereas bird sounds had the largest effect in reduction of physiological symptoms of stress and annoyance (blood pressure, pain reduction and heart rate). What also emerged was the fact that the complexity of natural sound also seems to be an important factor, with more complex natural sounds having significantly improved health and decreased levels of stress and annoyance, compared to fewer or no sounds.

But how important is hearing nature compared to seeing or smelling it? Teasing apart the relationship between these different senses and their relative importance is far from straightforward – especially outdoors when we are bombarded by all three. But it's an important question if we are considering using any of these sensory inputs, whether inside our homes or offices to try to induce calming or improved cognitive performance, or outside: how should we rank the environment that we choose to walk in to gain maximum health benefits via our different senses? Should it be a large open green space with scattered trees providing optimum visual stimulus; an area with fragrant plants doing us good through our sense of smell; or a woody copse or hedgerow with plentiful habitats for songbirds? I had always assumed that sight was most important. But studies looking into this question have totally challenged my preconceptions about the relative importance of hearing, seeing or smelling nature.

My first preconception was that seeing nature has more health benefits than hearing it. In fact, the opposite has now been found in several studies. For example, a study carried out by research scientists in Lund University in Sweden showed that we recover faster from stress when we *hear* sounds of nature compared to when we see it.[21] This study involved participants undergoing an induced stressful event (giving a speech and doing a maths test in front of an audience of three stony-faced actors) and then being placed in one of three 'recovery' rooms for fifteen minutes. One had nature sounds playing in the background (bird song and water), the other had scenes of the forest but with no sound, and the third had no sounds and plain walls. The fastest recovery from stress (as recorded in a number of physiological markers such as heart-rate variability, respiration rate and so on) occurred in those that heard the sounds of nature. In fact, those that just saw forest environments with no sound mentioned that they had experienced fear, expecting something threatening or dangerous to appear. Silent nature can be spooky.

However, a note of caution must be added here, since no differences were found in some of the physiological measures of stress (e.g. salivary cortisol). This may well be to do with the time-frame of the experiment; levels of cortisol are often slow to change in response to a stressor and may have occurred beyond the time-limit of the experiment. The authors themselves suggest that more studies are needed to determine the relative roles of hearing and seeing forest environments and their impact on physiological stress recovery.[22] But the overall take-home message remains strong – hearing nature is important for stress reduction.

But how does the influence of one sense stack up against the other two? Studies that have looked into the relative importance of sight, sound and smell on our health seem to indicate that a combination of all three types of sensory stimulus has the most significant impact, at least in reducing stress.

This is particularly well demonstrated by a study carried out by research scientists from the Swedish University of Agricultural Sciences.[23] They devised an experiment to examine the additional benefits obtained from hearing and smelling nature when added to existing natural visual stimulus. A large and mixed group of 154 participants took part. As with other studies cited in this book, their approach involved testing in a clinical setting how quickly participants recovered from an induced stressful situation. This time the stressor was mild electric shocks (not something I would rush to volunteer for myself). These were delivered through electrodes to the index and middle fingers on the non-dominant hand.

After the shocks were administered, physiological recovery rates from the deliberately raised levels of stress were measured using skin conductance tests, which were assessed continuously throughout the experiment. During recovery, participants were exposed to a variety of sensory stimuli in different combinations. All were shown a visual image, one of several 3D 360° virtual reality photos, featuring a densely built urban environment, a forest or an urban park. They also experienced various sounds and smells at the same time, including birdsong and traffic noise, and the smells of grass, fir, tar and diesel. They viewed and sensed these different experiences for five minutes after the one minute of electric shocks, and their stress recovery rates were measured during this time.

The findings were clear and statistically strong. Unsurprisingly, for the vast majority of participants, seeing the park and forest scenes led to significantly faster stress reduction compared to the urban scene. Importantly, however, stress recovery was faster when they also heard birdsong, and even more so when the grass smell was also included. In fact, when all three senses of nature were combined, this resulted in the fastest stress reduction recovery.

The authors concluded that parks and forests that include both the sounds of singing birds and natural smells should be prioritised in our daily lives since they can offer the fastest and most effective ways of lowering stress levels. The beneficial effects appear within minutes.[24] I would go further than this and suggest that we should take this into consideration for indoor environments as well. Good sounds are good for you.

But what about the opposite effect? If good sounds are good for us, how do we mitigate the negative health effects of bad sounds? Traffic, building sites, alarms and other noises are all around us, including in urban green spaces. Is there some sort of threshold level of bad noises that outweighs the beneficial sounds?

We already know that certain urban sounds carry negative health benefits.[25] Can the positive sounds of nature reduce some of these impacts? This is a difficult question to address because of the complexity of the types of sounds, their volume, variation and relation to each other within a city environment. It involves separating out urban and natural sounds from the overall soundscape, measuring both, and looking for a threshold point where the one sound masks the other.

So far I have found only one experiment addressing this question. Konrad Uebel and colleagues from the University of Queensland framed the question as a negative: at what point do traffic noises negate the benefits that we obtain from hearing nature?[26] They aimed to disentangle the effects of different sounds and identify where the threshold between good and bad responses occurs.

Uebel and his colleagues made a series of seventy-second recordings of soundscapes commonly experienced by park users within the Brisbane Local Government Area between 6.30 and 7.30 a.m., capturing different levels of bird activity and morning traffic noise volume. They then scaled the soundbites to describe their content. Bird sounds were given a score of 1 to 5, with 1 equalling very low presence of birdsong and 5 very high, within each. Traffic sound was scaled in decibels. This resulted in a selection of eight soundbites that provided a gradient of park soundscape samples, ranging from high traffic noise and very low bird activity to very low traffic noise and high bird activity.

Each participant listened to all eight soundbites in a laboratory, but in different orders to remove any bias. After listening they answered a series of questions based on their perception of the sound, how restorative it was and what they thought the effect of this restorative potential might be on their own feelings of well-being.

What emerged clearly was that those soundscapes where birds were louder and traffic noise was at its lowest were percceived to be most restorative. In contrast, as the traffic noise increased, the potential restorative effect of the bird sounds become more and more diminished. In effect they managed to develop a quantitatively sliding scale showing a threshold beyond which bad urban sounds start to destroy the benefits of good nature sounds.

These sorts of practical findings are important, particularly for city planners – but also for us. Where are the best places to walk to get maximum benefit from the sounds of nature? This requires some sort of sonic mapping system that balances out good and bad noise in the spaces within our urban environments.

This brings me to my final study of this chapter. A team of researchers from the Department of Sound at the University of Chile have attempted to do exactly this: to create maps depicting hotspots of good sound in city green spaces.[27]

First, they used results from existing studies, some of which are described above, to select the key sounds associated with positive mental health benefits. These they called health restoration soundscapes. They then further ranked these sounds by developing a scoring system within the category of sounds with an overall beneficial effect: for example, the volume of sound from anthropogenic sources had to be below 50 decibels to classify as good and gain a high score (the distant sound of children playing in a park can be delightfully soothing; living next door to a nursery or busy school playground can become wearing). They also had a similar sliding scale of marks for the composition of the perceived sound source (that is, whether it was mainly from natural, technological or human sounds – with natural sounds scoring higher), how busy the soundscape was (calm, vibrant or chaotic) and if one sense dominated the environment (smell, sound, sight). The total amount of 'naturalness' was also assessed as the percentage of ground covered by natural elements.

This scoring system was then applied to twenty-one urban green spaces in Argentina, Sweden and Chile, providing a quantitative metric to score them for the quality of their soundscapes. To score highly, aspects of all beneficial criteria had to be present to some degree. Worryingly, of these twenty-one urban green spaces in these contrasting cities, only three were found to contain soundscapes with the potential to offer health restoration effects: two in areas of the Stadsparken City Park in Lund, Sweden, and the University Botanic Garden in Valdivia, Chile.

So, we clearly have a lot of work to do. We need to improve our urban soundscapes. Science is telling us that, in sound as much as in sight and smell, nature is good for our physical and mental health. Good sounds help in relieving stress, restoring us and relieving our pain. Bad sounds don't. But this aspect gets far too little attention in the public policy field. Developers and applicants for planning permission are required to demonstrate how people will access green space, and make commitments to things like biodiversity net gain and connectivity. But they are not required to measure and consider the sonic environment, at least not to anything like a sufficient degree. Too many people live too close to noisy roads, without adequate sonic protection being required by law. Depressingly, this is still often the case with new-build developments. We are storing up trouble. The rapid move towards electric cars and buses will certainly help by making traffic quieter, but the really big, noisy vehicles on our roads, like lorries, are not there yet in terms of technology.

We can help ourselves, too. Be aware of the sounds around you and choose to spend time with the good ones. Walk to work through the park or a quiet urban street where you can hear birdsong. If it adds a few more minutes to your commute – great: they'll be the best minutes you'll have all day.

We need to allow nature to sing to us.

6

The Proven Health Benefits of Tree-Hugging

Recently I found myself walking around the Botanic Garden in Oxford. This beautiful and historic location, right in the heart of the city, attracts over 200,000 visitors a year to its tranquil walkways and restful vistas.

But it wasn't just the elegant variety of plants, or even the impressive range of the scientific research being undertaken here, that caught my attention. It was a small child reaching out to touch the leaf of a rose, and her grandmother, instead of telling her not to touch, stroking the silky petal against her cheek. The child was intrigued and delighted.

We are often told, 'Don't Touch' and 'Keep Off The Grass'. Maybe it's time to ditch those outdated attitudes. Maybe experiencing nature through the medium of tactile interaction with leaves, bark and petals is good for us. Maybe Grandma was right.

The urge to touch things is one we have from a very early age. Take a toddler into a shop, and they simply have to touch everything in sight. This is because we use touch to learn. But is there a deeper significance to our response to how nature feels, as well as to how it looks, sounds and smells?

A few years ago, the idea of allowing animals into hospital wards, nursing homes and children's vaccination clinics would have been unthinkable. The risk of infection would have been regarded as too great. Times have changed. When I recently visited an old relative in a care home, the room was full of dogs being stroked by the residents. It was clear from both the senior citizens' faces, and the dogs' wagging tails, that there was a joint 'love-in' going on. The happiness and mental well-being that stroking these dogs was bringing to the residents was clear to see – and it also made it clear to me why it is increasingly common to see therapy dogs in clinical environments. The positive emotions and reduced fear and anxiety that occurs when touching and stroking these dogs are now often deemed to outweigh the risks associated with their potential biohazard.[1] Interestingly, these studies are also revealing that individuals who engage in more physical contact with the dogs during these interactions show lower stress levels afterwards, suggesting that it may well be this element of tactile stimulation (touch) which provides the benefits we typically associate with being around animals.

But does the same thing work with inanimate nature? Can we derive similar benefits from touching leaves, stroking the bark of trees or even the timber of the trees, plant material that is long since dead?

Many of us certainly seem to have an instinctive wish, even need, to stroke the surfaces of wooden furniture – as beautifully illustrated in a conversation I had with Barnaby Scott, a local furniture maker in Oxfordshire who founded the company Waywood:

When people see my furniture, the first thing they ask is whether they can touch it, they're diffident, but we're all strongly drawn to touching wood and it is reassuringly warm.

And from the conversation it was clear that it is not just his customers that feel this way:

Wood provides a warm, reassuring environment with lovely associations from the living world, which other materials don't. When the workshop was asked to cut some plastic fence rails, we couldn't wait to get rid of them and return to our wood – the difference for everyone was palpable.

But what actually happens to us when we touch and stroke plant material? Does it invoke some of the same physiological and psychological calming mechanisms that occur when we stroke and touch certain animals? Should we hug trees in the park with the same lack of self-consciousness with which we pet our neighbour's cat?

It has been known for a long time that gardening is associated with many positive health benefits for young and old. Horticultural therapy is now a well-recognised occupational health intervention for those with mental health conditions such as depression and memory loss, particularly older people.[2] It has also been shown to be effective at reducing some of the chronic symptoms in patients with schizophrenia, and reducing stress levels and agitation in children with Attention Deficient Hyperactivity Disorder and autism.[3] It is often assumed that 'being outside' will do the trick by providing the combined benefits of sound, sight, smell, exercise and social interaction. This is probably correct – it is a combination of them all. But what specific role does touch play in this? Can we isolate its effects from our other senses? For example, therapeutic animal petting sessions often take place indoors without the additional environmental stimuli of the smells and sounds of nature or increased exercise. Are there specific changes that are triggered in our bodies when we touch plants?

One intriguing experiment that started me on this journey of questioning whether touching plants has an impact on our physical and mental well-being was one in which participants sat in a clinical environment with their eyes closed and were asked to touch four different materials: a leaf of a living pothos plant (*Epipremnum aureum*, which we have met already under its alternative name, devil's ivy); an artificial pothos leaf made from resin; a piece of soft fabric; and a metal plate. While doing so they had their brain scanned using infrared spectroscopy in order to detect changes in cerebral blood flow and therefore central nervous system activity.[4] Clear results emerged: touching the living leaf of the pothos plant resulted in a significant calming response compared to touching the other materials.

This was a simple experiment with a small number or participants – just fourteen. But, for me, it raised other questions – not least, how common are these sorts of responses when we touch and stroke plant material such as the different types of wood, or the leaves on a living plant? Also, which parts of our bodies should be doing the touching; is it just touching with our hands, or do we get a similar response when, for example, we walk barefoot on grass or wooden floors? These experiences are often part of our daily lives; are they actually doing us good? Should we actively seek them out?

We each have millions of receptors which respond to various touch stimuli distributed throughout our skin. However, certain parts of our bodies – our face and hands, for example – have a much higher density of these receptors. This explains why these areas are much more receptive to external physical stimuli, including touch. There are also several different kinds of receptors in our skin, stimulated by mechanical touch (stroking, stretching, vibration), temperature (thermoreceptors) and chemicals (chemoreceptors). Our skin, muscle, joints and most of our internal organs also contain pain receptors (nociceptors) that are activated by actions that potentially damage tissue. When we touch something, these receptors are activated and generate signals which travel along sensory nerves to neurons in the spinal cord and to the thalamus region in the brain. The neurons in the thalamus region then relay signals to other parts of the brain that trigger a variety of different responses including, for example, movement of our limbs, change in our heart rate, respiration rate, attention, focus and awareness. This is the practical, physical response to the stimuli provided by the biology of touch.

It seems reasonable, therefore, to expect that touching plant material could invoke a response that is linked to health and well-being, but that, in some cases, a response might be at odds with those triggered by other senses. For example, Chapter 2 suggested that looking at bright green foliage might well invoke physiological calming. But plants that have this leaf colour include the poison ivy leaf (*Toxicodendron radicans*), touching which will result in a very different response, causing pain and an increase in physiological stress. We soon learn not to touch certain plants. Fortunately, this is not the case with most plants that we encounter in our daily lives. Most are harmless to touch. They offer a huge variety of tactile experience from the amazing diversity of surface texture: rough, smooth, shiny, waxy, or covered in soft hairs, needles, knots and protrusions.

We probably most often touch plant material not outside in a natural setting but in our homes and workspaces, making contact with wooden surfaces with our hands and our feet in the form of flooring, structural support such as beams, decorations like panelling, or furniture. What we are actually touching here is the inside parts of the tree trunk, known as the cambium and heartwood – material that has often taken between 40 and 120 years to develop before it is harvested for timber production.

The main distinction in the types of timber that we will encounter in our everyday lives is between so-called 'hardwoods' and 'softwoods'. Hardwoods are likely to be found in furniture and floorings where durability is important, while softwoods are used predominantly in timber, medium-density fibreboard (MDF), paper and for building components such as windows and doors. These terms are used by those working with wood as a product. For example, the briefest internet search of the term 'hardwood' offers me a large range of different types of flooring, compared to 'softwood', which offers me timber for garden decking and kitchen cabinets. However, what is probably less well known is that the vast majority of hardwoods are from angiosperm trees, whereas softwoods are from gymnosperm trees. These are the two most important groups in the plant kingdom.

The angiosperms are flowering plants and are distinguished by the fact that they produce seeds that are enclosed in an outer structure called an ovule, such as a fleshy fruit or nut. Flowering trees whose hardwood is often used for floors and furniture include cherry trees, oak, birch, beech and ash. Softwood in comparison comes from trees in the gymnosperm group, containing all the coniferous families including pine, fir, cypress and araucaria: the ones whose olfactory properties we discussed in Chapter 5. Their seeds are not encased in an outer covering but are 'naked' within an open structure such as a cone. The seeds of pine trees, for example (which, confusingly, are usually referred to as pine nuts in cooking), sit at the base of the scales of the cone and are released when it opens. Common gymnosperm trees used in timber production include pine, fir, spruce and larch.

But why do gymnosperms produce softwood and angiosperms hardwood? This is because there is a fundamental difference in the cells in the trunks which transport water and nutrients around the tree. Gymnosperm trees have one type of cell called a tracheid, which carries both water and nutrients. Their wood therefore appears uniform in cross-section and has a consistent sponge-like structure that is not very dense and not that good at heavy load-bearing, because it will compress and change shape fairly easily. In contrast, angiosperm wood contains two different types of cells in the tree trunk, one for transporting water (xylem), and the other for transporting nutrients (phloem) around the tree. These two cell types show up in the cross-section of the trunk as pores and holes of varying size. This complexity and arrangement of different cell sizes and shapes within the trunk makes the wood of the angiosperm much denser and more compact, and therefore stronger and better able to withstand external loads – hence the name hardwood.

Another difference between angiosperm and gymnosperm wood is its knottiness. Hardwood timber tends to contain a lot more knots than softwood because of the different branching structure of these two groups of trees. The next time you look at a beech, oak or ash tree (in the angiosperm group) compare the shape and arrangement of its branches on its trunk to those on a conifer such as pine and spruce (in the gymnosperm group). You will notice that conifers tend to have straight branches, small in diameter, often at right angles to the stem and more often than not located towards the top of the tree. In comparison, the branches of angiosperm trees such as oak, beech and ash have branches located almost at random throughout the stem, of many different sizes, diameters and shapes. Knots in the wood indicate where the branches were attached to the main trunk. So, this difference in branching structure means that softwoods have fewer knots, and the ones that are present are smaller and more regularly spaced, while hardwoods have lots of knots of different shapes and sizes, which often appear to be randomly distributed across the wood.

These features certainly affect how easy each type is to work with. But do they have any impact on our response when we touch them? Few researchers have to date asked this question. However, a novel study carried out over ten years ago by a team of scientists from the Shizuoka Industrial Research Institute, Japan, was one of the first to indicate that there may indeed be differences in our response to different kinds of timber.[5] This took the form of an experiment in a clinical setting where participants touched pieces of softwood (Japanese hinoki cypress, *Chamaecyparis obtusa*, and Japanese cedar, *Cryptomeria japonica*), hardwood (oak, known as mizunara, *Quercus crispula)* and two manufactured materials (aluminium and acrylic plastic). The materials were all at the same temperature, and the participants were instructed to keep their eyes closed to isolate the effect of touch from other sensory inputs. During the experiment blood pressure and pulse rate were measured every second. Participants also completed a sensory evaluation immediately after touching each material.

The most obvious and perhaps unsurprising finding was a clear difference in response between touching manufactured materials and touching wood. Touching the manufactured material increased blood pressure and pulse rate. Participants also reported a negative sensory experience compared to touching wood. However, more intriguing was the second finding that there were also clear differences in response between the species of wood.

Touching hardwood produced a rise in blood pressure, whereas touching the softwoods led to no significant change. In addition, participants rated the sensory experience of touching softwood as safe and comfortable.

This relatively simple experiment suggests that tactile interaction with wood may lead to calming, and that this effect may be species specific. I say 'may' and caution must be expressed here because the sample size was very small, the parameters (physiological and psychological) measured were few, and this is just one experiment. I was therefore ready to dismiss it as providing insufficient evidence until I came across several later experiments, examining more physiological and psychological parameters, and finding the same sorts of results. For example, in an experiment carried out by Professor Harumi Ikei and colleagues from the University of Chiba in 2018, they found significant physiological and psychological differences in participants when they touched oak wood compared to surfaces of marble, clay and stainless steel.[6] These included differences in brain activity, heart-rate variability and mood profiles. While touching the four different materials the participants were blindfolded so they couldn't see what they were touching. They touched each material with the palm of their hand and the materials were at the same temperature. What emerged was a clear indication that touching white oak in comparison to the other three materials resulted in physiological relaxation. The self-evaluation mood questionnaire also indicated psychological relaxation (lower tension-anxiety scores) after touching white oak compared to other materials.[7] Sadly in this experiment they didn't also touch a softwood – but this would certainly be an interesting next step.

But does this only work when we touch a material with our hands? This matters, since we often experience a surface in other ways, for example through our feet when walking on a wooden floor. To address this Ikei's team set up a follow-on experiment, using the same suite of techniques to measure physiological stress and psychological responses as previously, but this time with the participants touching the materials with their feet.[8] Another difference from the first experiment is that this time the softwood species Hinokicypress (*Chamaecyparis obtusa*) was used. The comparison material was marble. Again, the results clearly indicated that touching wood with the soles of the feet induced physiological and psychological relaxation compared to the marble. In the questionnaire, respondents used words such as 'relaxed', 'comfortable' and 'natural' to describe the sensation of being in contact with wood, as opposed to terms like 'indifferent' and 'slightly uncomfortable' for the sensation of touching marble.

For me, this suggests that it is time to ditch the shoes and walk around barefoot in rooms with wooden floors. However, most wood we touch has been smoothed and treated with oil, varnish, wax or polish, giving a wide variety of different feels and finishes, known to the trade as 'vitreous', 'mirror' and other terms. Varnish, for example, tends to smooth out natural roughness, and sanding makes natural knots, ridges and furrows much less prominent. So, do these treatments and changes to the surface texture influence our responses to it?

Some of the first researchers to ask this question were not medical scientists but rather those involved in designing furniture, who were keen to understand people's preferences for different finishes of items such as kitchen cabinets and worktops. I often stroke the surface of a cabinet, table or other furniture when looking to buy it, yet I never think about this role of touch playing any part in my decision-making process. But if the experiments by Shiv Bhatta and colleagues from the University of Helsinki are anything to go by, it clearly does. They asked participants to touch surfaces of softwood (Scots pine – *Pinus sylvestris*) and hardwood (oak – *Quercus robur*) that had been sanded with sandpaper, or brushed with a metal brush, or coated with double layer varnish, or waxed. They also touched wooden boards covered with silk cloth and sandpaper. During the experiment the participants were seated in a temperature-controlled room and unable to see the material that they were touching, and they were asked to run their fingertip back and forth over each material for eight seconds, which is probably similar to the length of time that most of us take to make an initial assessment of a material through touch. The order of touching the different materials was randomly assigned between participants to reduce any bias. After touching each material they filled in a questionnaire on their sensory and emotional perception of the different finishes.[9]

Even with this relatively simple experiment, the participants' preferences for the different surface-treatments were remarkably aligned. Natural wood surfaces (no wax or varnish) were rated significantly higher in all the descriptors that featured positive emotional ratings in comparison to the coated wood surfaces. Additionally, the natural surfaces were rated least irritating and uncomfortable in the descriptors that featured the negative aspects of touch.

It would therefore appear that the naturalness of the surface properties of wood-based products may be linked to positive perceptions of the material.[10] Interestingly, returning to the conversation with Barnaby Scott, it would appear that even a seasoned furniture maker has different feelings according to how the wood is treated: 'I instinctively felt drawn to wood and have always favoured solid wood even to a veneer. There's a friendliness and warmth to a solid piece of elm or oak, which is lovely to touch, you can feel the hollow bundles in their grain. There's a joy in it.'

But does this preference and perception lead to actual physiological changes in our bodies? As crazy as it might at first sound, it would appear we do have a different physiological response when we touch untreated wood, compared to other finishes. For example, when researchers examined the brain activity and heart-rate variability of participants while they were touching plates of uncoated, oil-finished, vitreous-finished, urethane-finished and mirror-finished white oak wood, even after only ninety seconds, there were clear differences in the participants' stress responses.[11] Uncoated wood led to more physiological calming, with a gradation apparent in the types of treated wood and their impact; oil and vitreous wood finishes were more calming compared to mirror-finished wood.

These few studies, showing that we experience physiological and psychological calming when touching wood with our hands and feet, were a real revelation to me. While a lot more work is clearly needed in this research area, they strongly hint that touching certain aspects of nature might have many beneficial health outcomes. But what they also made me curious to explore was how much we currently know about touching live plant material such as stems and leaves, particularly when working in gardens and tending our houseplants. We already know that gardening has many physical and mental health benefits associated with it (discussed in later chapters) – but how much of this can be attributed to actively touching the plants?

There are still only a few experiments to date that ask the specific question: what happens when we touch plant stems and leaves? Those that have are usually coming at this from a different angle – while inadvertently answering this question in the process. For example, one such experiment aimed to see if children gained more benefits from playing with real plants compared to playing a horticultural game with plants on their mobile phone. Given what is known about the benefits in just seeing green plants, even on a screen or in a picture (see Chapters 2 and 3), it would not be unreasonable to expect that playing plant games on a computer screen should carry the same sort of benefits as the real thing; however this is not what the researchers found.[12]

Both experiments occurred indoors (i.e. where other factors could not also influence responses). The real gardening activity involved taking stem cuttings from a plant and then planting them in pots filled with soil. In comparison the gardening activity on the mobile phone was a game simulating a realistic environment in which the children could select seeds and grow them in a virtual world. While carrying out these two tasks, four measures were taken to detect physiological and psychological changes in the children: heart-rate variability, skin conductance, skin temperature, and levels of mood and anxiety recorded in self-reporting questionnaires. Each activity was carried out for five minutes with breaks between them and the order of the tasks varied to ensure that other factors such as tiredness were not influencing the outcome.

Strongly significant results emerged: when playing with real plants the children were much more physiologically relaxed compared to the horticultural mobile phone game activity. They also reported feeling more comfortable and cheerful, and their anxiety scores were significantly lower after the horticultural task compared to the mobile phone game task, suggesting that psychological calming was occurring as well. In the conclusion to this study, the lead author, Yuhan Shao, neatly summarised the practical implications of this finding, saying that 'engagement of children in horticultural activities in school could reduce stress and promote their physiological and psychological relaxation'.[13]

Given this finding, it is good therefore to see outdoor gardening activities becoming part of the routine school curricula in some countries, as is certainly the case in the UK. The only downside is that these require space outside and funding to operate, and this is a reason these indoor studies are so encouraging, because they suggest that even touching plant material in a classroom can invoke physiological and psychological calming. This finding is also pleasing for any of us who spend some time each day tending our houseplants, an activity which often involves touching the leaves.

Thinking about my own domestic routines, however, made me wonder if touching our plants also has any impact on our cognitive function. I say this because I have a habit of tending my plants when I am seeking a mental break from other tasks (especially writing – never have my houseplants looked so pristine as when I was writing this book). So, does this activity of touching plants act as a mini mental break and increase our focus, or is it just a distraction? As yet there are very few studies looking at this question, and we must remember that even seeing green plants has been shown to act as a mini mental break and improve accuracy of cognitively demanding tasks (see Chapter 1). But one study I came across involving children and measuring their brain activity while carrying out a number of different touching tasks, including one involving leaves and stems of plants, made me wonder whether there is indeed something further to be gained by touching as well as viewing green plants.[14]

This study involved eleven-year-olds carrying out various horticultural activities including planting seeds, mixing soils and harvesting plants, and non-horticultural activities such as playing with a ball, paper folding, reading, watching videos and solving maths problems during a seventy-minute time window. Each child carried out all activities but in different orders to remove any effect of tiredness influencing the result, with each task lasting for three minutes.

While doing them, their brain activity was measured with electrodes placed on specific regions of the children's scalp in order to record activity in the prefrontal lobes of the brain. This is the part that plays an important role in attention, working memory and goal-orientated behaviour.

The results were fascinating and showed that the simple activity of harvesting lettuces, which involved touching the leaves and stems when selecting and cutting them from a tray, showed the greatest change in brain activity in the prefrontal lobes.[15] Other activities involving touching other organic material, such as seeds and soils, did not show the same effect, suggesting that it was handling the leafy plant material that was associated with the improved cognitive abilities. Although this is a small sample size and these results must therefore be treated as preliminary, it hints that as well as inducing calming, the action of touching plants may make us more focused and attentive.

Having reviewed current research on touching plants, I think it is fair to say that our knowledge on touch is still a long way behind that associated with our other senses and this is backed up by quantitative data on this matter. For example, a recent analysis of studies published between 2008 and 2018 on the different senses and their influence on mental well-being found over 1,500 research articles on sight compared to just 40 on touch.[16]

Two reasons have traditionally been put forward for this research bias. First, that vision is perceived as more important than other senses because is it the main way we interact with the world. Second, the processing of visual information is far more complex and occupies larger parts of our brain than the processing of sensory information from other senses and therefore warrants greater research effort.

These inferences are not without their critics, however. Some have recently suggested that this bias is also technological and cultural. Specifically, present-day technology is better suited for studying vision than other senses, giving it greater prominence in research. And discussion and language around vision has almost always given it a dominant role among the senses in Western societies.[17] Two thousand years ago, Plato was one of the first to give vision the greatest emphasis among the senses, even referring to it as 'divine' in one instance. Aristotle's view was a little more nuanced: while he says that touch is our gateway to the palpable properties of the elements, vision is the highest sense for the natural philosopher. He even created a hierarchy, putting vision first, followed by hearing, smell, taste and touch. Aristotle's insights remained influential, if not always accepted in their entirety, essentially right up until today. Interestingly, this primacy of the visual sense in written texts does not appear to be the case in all non-Western cultures: while English has comparatively more words for things we can see, there are some cultures whose languages have a bias toward touch (for example Dogul Dom, spoken in Mali, and Siwu, spoken in Ghana).[18]

Further research into the effects of our sense of touch is therefore needed, including on how varied our responses are according to different types of leaves and wood, and if the age, gender and culture of the people doing the touching affects the outcome. Also, we need to determine how long the benefits will last once the tactile stimulation is removed. We know, for example, that some of the benefits associated with interacting with nature through our sense of smell, such as elevated natural killer cells in our blood, can last for days (see Chapter 4). I am assuming this is not the case with touching plants – but it would be good to understand better the frequency with which we need to touch our houseplants, or stroke our wooden tables, to gain maximum benefits.

Another thing we need to be mindful about when researching touch is that while touching plants may benefit us, it doesn't always benefit the plant. An experiment looking at the effects of human touch on mouse-ear cress (*Arabidopsis thaliana*), for example, showed that even the slightest touch activated a major genetic defence response which, if repeated, could significantly impact its growth: plants that were touched were significantly shorter twelve weeks later than those that weren't.[19] In addition, some plants are not good for us to touch because they have a defence mechanism to prevent them being eaten. An obvious example is the stinging nettle (*Urtica dioica*). This species has its stems and leaves covered by delicate hollow hair-like structures called trichomes, which contain a chemical cocktail of histamine, acetylcholine and serotonin that causes inflammation and pain. When you touch this plant, the fragile silica tips are broken off these hairs and they act like needles, piercing and injecting the chemical cocktail into your skin, causing the familiar stinging sensation and a rash. For the good of both parties, therefore, it is important to know which plants are good to touch and which are not.

A final point to note relating to the touching experiments is that many of them do not isolate the sense of sight from touch. This is particularly true of those involving gardening activities as one of the tasks – which for obvious reasons needs people to be able to see what they are doing when using sharp tools to cut and transplant plants. Further work is therefore required to tease these senses of sight and touch apart. In the meantime, a pragmatic view is that both seeing and touching green plants appears to reduce our levels of stress and anxiety and improve our mental focus.

Armed with this evidence, I am now off to tend my houseplants.

7

Hidden Senses

Whenever I give a public talk about the health benefits associated with sensing nature, there is always a question from someone in the audience about the things we can't see, hear, smell or touch but are known to exist all around us – environmental microbes.

Given the surge in knowledge over the past decade about the microbiota of our gut, and how the millions of microbes (mainly bacteria) that exist in it can have a profound positive impact on our health, I assume this is what is driving these questions: if these microbes do so much good in our gut, what about those that are found in the natural environment around us – do they provide us with any health benefits?

I have to admit (somewhat ashamedly) to previously stating that the environmental microbiome did not really have any direct impact on our health. How wrong could I be? This chapter will tell you just how wrong. In my defence, our scientific understanding of its full potential for our health is only now emerging. Having now read that emerging science, I have become a total convert.

I believe that this area of research represents some of the most exciting and potentially important evidence for a strong biological link to the natural environmental microbiome and explains why we should all spend a lot more time interacting with nature, both outdoors and indoors.

I was first introduced to this emerging area of science by Professor Gretchen Daily from Stanford University. She mentioned a research project conducted in Finland that showed how letting kindergarten-aged children play in a yard that contained 'dirt' from the forest floor compared to manufactured materials (for example plastics and concrete) resulted in a significant and positive impact on their gut microbiome. Published in 2020 in a top scientific journal, *Science Advances*, the study set up an experiment with children in kindergartens, typically aged between three and five years old, to see what happened to their skin and gut microbiomes and their immune system function if they played in areas containing elements of nature.[1] Seventy-nine young children took part, all living in urban environments and spending the majority of their days at different daycare centres around Finland. The only difference between them was that these daycare centres had three different types of outdoor spaces. The first was a fairly standard outdoor play area, comprised of concrete, gravel and some plastic matting. The second was the type typically found in daycare environments that are already nature-orientated: these have grass, soil and planted areas for the children to play in. They are usually at the top end in terms of price and therefore not that common – at least in the UK. These two acted as a control against which to compare the results from the third experimental space type. In the experimental areas, the concrete and gravel were covered with segments of forest floor and soil from the local coniferous forest. Planters for growing plants and peat blocks for climbing and digging were also introduced into these spaces.

The children were encouraged to play in only one of the three types of yard each day over the twenty-eight days of the experiment. Before and after periods of play, the children's skin and gut microbiota were measured using genetic sequencing of the bacteria taken from skin swabs and stool samples, along with changes in their blood for immunoregulatory cytokine levels and T_{reg} cell frequencies. These cells and proteins play a critical role in preventing autoimmunity and autoimmune diseases; their levels in our blood are often used as an indication of how well the immune system is functioning. Remarkable results emerged. After the study concluded, the children who played in the experimental yard showed a large increase in the diversity of microbiota on their skin and in their gut in comparison to the children playing in the urban and nature-orientated areas. Importantly, these were the 'good' types of microbiota (i.e. those known to be associated with many health benefits).[2] There was also a significant increase in the children's blood markers, indicative of them having gained enhanced immunoregulatory pathways – which itself is indicative of a reduced risk of immune-mediated diseases such as inflammatory bowel disease and rheumatoid arthritis.

The importance of this study cannot be overstated. It implies that even short-term exposure to nature's microbial diversity has the potential to radically alter the diversity of microbiota on our skin and in our gut. In addition, it suggests that the altered gut microbiota can modulate the function of our immune system.[3] I found this extraordinary – that something in the natural environment that we cannot see, smell, hear or touch, yet becomes incorporated into our bodies, can trigger a set of changes in our gut that can influence our immune system function and associated health. I wanted to know more, starting with an understanding of what the human microbiome is all about.

When people talk about the human microbiome they are normally referring to the microbes that exist in our gut (the gastrointestinal part of our bodies), on our skin and in our respiratory tract, even though, as you can imagine, these tiny organisms are found in and on all parts of our body. Our gut in particular contains an incredibly abundant and diverse microbial community of more than 100 trillion microorganisms. In fact, our colon is so microbially diverse that it is estimated to be one of the most populated habitats on Earth.[4] Whereas the microbiome is the term used to describe the whole community, it is the microbiota, the individual groups within it, that are the most important to understand. These include bacteria, yeasts and viruses – but by a long way, bacteria are the dominant player with around 90 per cent of our gut microbiome thought to be made up of them. It is the functions they perform, and the compounds that they produce, that trigger responses in other organs including our heart, kidney, blood vessels and even our brain.[5]

The role of these microbiota communities in our gut is now thought to be so significant that it is often referred to as a super-organism, considered alongside the heart, lungs and brain in terms of its importance to our health. For example, our own organs can only synthesise eleven of the twenty essential amino acids that we need to obtain from food, so the remaining nine, along with thirteen essential vitamins, are retrieved and synthesised by the microbes in our gut. Many microbes also produce a large variety of chemicals known as secondary metabolites, which include some of the most important compounds for our health including immuno-suppressants, anti-cancer and anti-inflammatory compounds.[6]

Everyone has a distinctive community of microbes in their gut, and this first develops when we are born. In the first few days, weeks and years of our life, the microbiota in our gut are strongly influenced by a number of external factors including birth age (pre-term babies, for example, show a low diversity of gut microbes and an increased level of potentially dangerous bacteria), type of delivery (natural birth versus caesarean), methods of milk feeding and weaning period. However, by the time we are about three years old, we all have a 'grown-up' microbiome in our gut – that is, the composition and diversity are most like those of an adult.

Despite containing many different types of microbiota, over 90 per cent of our gut microbiota fall into one of five dominant groups.[7] This gut microbial composition stays relatively stable until we reach old age. Having said this, over time distinct differences are apparent both within and between individuals relating to a variety of factors. A person's ethnicity, the food they consume, antibiotic use, body size and the amount of exercise they take each day all leave a clear signature on their gut microbial diversity. In fact, the differences in these gut microbiota are so clear that in some cases, a person's traits, such as their glycaemic response to eating certain foods, can be predicted from their gut microbiota alone.

What I find interesting and important in relation to our gut microbiome is the fact that these microbial communities don't just help our gut extract nutrients from food. Rather, they appear to be associated with the functioning of our immune system, central nervous system and associated health outcomes: so much so that people's microbiomes significantly differ in microbial composition – and clear correlations have been found between particular gut microbiota (so called 'sick' microbiomes) and certain illnesses.[8] Those illnesses with a distinctive gut microbial signature include intestinal disorders such as irritable bowel syndrome, inflammatory bowel disease, celiac disease and colorectal cancer as well as non-intestinal disorders such as obesity and type 2 diabetes. In addition, illnesses related to the central nervous system such as Alzheimer's and Parkinson's diseases, hepatic encephalopathy (psychiatric abnormalities in patients with liver dysfunction), autism spectrum disorders and even stress, depression and hypertension also demonstrate distinctive signature gut microbial communities.[9]

Even though it is relatively early days in terms of understanding how these gut–brain health interactions work, recognising that there is a link between the health of our gut microbiome and these illnesses is an important discovery. What is even more remarkable is the discovery that our environment (broadly defined – meaning, diet, lifestyle, antibiotic use and so on) appears to have a stronger influence on our gut microbiome than our genetic background.[10] In fact, less than 8 per cent of our gut composition is now thought to be due to genetic inheritance; the rest is due to our lifestyle and the environment.[11] The implications of this are profound, because it suggests that by changing our environment and hence gut microbiota from a 'sick' to a 'healthy' composition, we may be able to prevent and/ or improve certain debilitating illnesses. But this then prompts the question: how do we go about changing our gut microbiota for the better? This is where a whole new area of research is emerging.

There are now at least nine different approaches being proposed by the medical profession and others as potentially important interventions to improve the diversity and communities of good microbiota in our gut microbiome, and thereby our health.[12] Some are more medically intrusive than others, but all, to some degree, have been shown in clinical trials to bring about marked improvements in microbial gut composition.[13]

What I think anyone would classify as clinically intrusive methods include, for example faecal transplants. As the name suggests, this involves taking stools (poo) from individuals with good gut microbiota for a specific health condition, and transplanting it, or some modified form of it, into the person that lacks these essential microbes. There is also phage therapy, which involves giving patients viruses known to target certain 'bad' or at least 'less useful' bacteria in the gut, which theoretically will then allow the more useful ones to flourish.

Easier, and probably more palatable, non-clinical interventions shown to have some success include making changes to our lifestyle, such as eating a diet more typical of that eaten in the Mediterranean region. This includes eating more fruit, nuts, vegetables, fish, chicken and olive oil and moving away from processed foods, refined sugars and most red meat. Meat and vegetables should also be organically grown, if possible, or at least washed extremely well before consumption. This is because there is alarming evidence to show that agriculture uses about four times more antibiotics than human medicine.[14] Antibiotics that are fed to cattle (in many regions of the world cattle are routinely given antibiotics as a precaution against disease) pass into our gut when we eat the meat and can have the same effect on our gut microbiota as if we had taken them ourselves, killing off many of the good microbiota. And this is not only the case for meat: these antibiotics are also found in the animal's faeces, which are then used as a fertiliser and sprayed onto crops – which we then eat.

Eating fermented foods such as sauerkraut is also shown to make a significant positive difference to our gut microbiota. The same is true for supplements (pre-, pro- and post-biotic concoctions) that are specifically constructed to contain high quantities of 'good' microbiota.[15] These include, for example, products that can be purchased in drinking form and/or added to other products such as kefir, 'live' yoghurts and probiotic drinks.

Since this knowledge on the importance of the gut microbiome has emerged, there has been a mushrooming of articles, books, potions and drugs to help us change our gut microbiota for the better. Yet possibly one of the most important actions, and still missing from many of these sources of advice, is simply for us to interact more with nature and its associated environmental microbiome – especially when some of this evidence now suggests that interacting with nature-derived microbiota could in fact be far more useful and effective than taking orally administered probiotics. But what type of nature-derived microbiota are we talking about, and what are the health benefits that we might expect to gain from interacting with its environmental microbiome?

The term 'environmental biome' refers to the microbiota associated with plants and soils and in the air around them. Like us, all terrestrial plants and soils are inhabited by a diverse, complex and interactive community of microorganisms. These microbiomes play an essential role in nutrient uptake and growth in plants, improving resilience against pathogens and sustaining plant growth under stress.[16] However, probably most interesting (and often unknown) in relation to human health, is the fact that the microbiomes of plants and soil share very similar bacteria communities to our own, being composed of five major bacterial phyla that are also found in the human gut and skin. Also similar to our situation is the way that healthy and sick microbiomes in plants and soil can change in positive or negative ways due to external environmental factors – organic soil, for example, containing a good diverse microbiome can greatly improve plant growth and health. Conversely, the addition of inorganic fertilisers, herbicides and so on can greatly reduce the diversity of soil and plant microbiota.

So why is spending time in the environmental microbiome so important? Because when we do, new evidence suggests it passes onto our skin and into our gut through ingestion and greatly improves our own gut microbiota and associated health benefits. This environmental microbiome hypothesis (called the 'biodiversity hypothesis') was first proposed over two decades ago in one of those papers that should be read by everyone, particularly people involved with managing urban green spaces around the world. Sadly, however, I fear that outside of academia this hypothesis has largely passed under the radar. The authors, Leena von Hertzen and Tari Haahtela, medical scientists at the Helsinki University Central Hospital, and Ilkka Hanski, a biodiversity scientist in the Helsinki Department of Biosciences, suggested that by spending time in and around naturally biodiverse environments, we increase the diversity of microbiota in our own bodies.[17] With this increase we gain a larger and more diverse arsenal of microbiota better able to deal with day-to-day digestive functions, and protection from various health conditions, particularly autoimmune diseases. They also suggested that the apparently close association between the loss of global biodiversity and the rise in immune dysfunction and disease provides evidence that the two are connected. By losing microbial diversity, which goes hand in hand with biodiversity loss, we have lost the important protection that it provides to our bodies against allergy and other autoimmune diseases.

Of course, this is only a hypothesis, and the apparent declines in biodiversity and rise in allergies are a correlation and do not necessarily indicate causation. But the significance of this paper cannot be overestimated. It proposes a clear and testable hypothesis – and is in line with other similar hypotheses relating to the importance of microbial diversity for our health which have since been shown to be broadly correct. For example, the 'hygiene

Association between biodiversity and public health

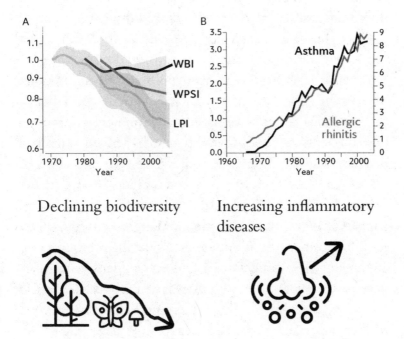

Declining biodiversity

Increasing inflammatory diseases

Source: L. Von Hertzen, I. Hanski and T. Haahtela.

hypothesis', which posits that living in environments that are too clean, often found in the developed world, robs infants of the necessary challenges to develop strong immune systems. The hygiene hypothesis is often used when discussing the high rates of asthma in the developed world. Conversely, it is widely accepted that environments that are rich in microbial diversity, in the home, in food, drinking water and on domestic animals, confers protection against allergic and autoimmune diseases. The biodiversity hypothesis is in effect an extension of this – suggesting that we should also interact with the natural environment because of the importance of nature-derived microbial diversity.

Over the past twenty years, a series of studies have set out to test this biodiversity hypothesis. To do this, however, has required testing three 'sub-hypotheses' or assumptions. The first is that there are significant differences between the microbial diversity of natural environments and urban environments. Second, that this nature-derived microbial diversity transfers into our bodies when we are close to nature, and this alters our own microbiota. Third, that the presence of nature-derived microbial diversity in our bodies triggers changes in our immune and allergic pathways, which result in positive health outcomes. Achieving robust data on all three of these is a tall order, and no wonder twenty years have passed since the hypothesis was first proposed. It is also fair to say that this is still an emerging field. However, the science, especially in the last decade or so, is getting to the point where leading microbiologists, such as Graham Rook from University College London, are now stating that this hypothesis is probably broadly correct, and that interacting with environmental microbial diversity, a hidden sense of nature, could be very important for the regulation of our immune system and associated diseases.[18]

The first assumption to be proved broadly correct was that there are significant differences in microbial diversity and abundance between natural environments and urban ones. While large-scale global analysis of environmental microbiomes associated with different nature regions of the world are yet to be undertaken, a handful of local and regional studies are revealing clear differences in the diversity and abundance of microbial communities both outdoors and indoors. Using genetic tools to identify the bacterial communities present, microbial diversity has been measured 'in the air, soil and on the leaves of plants across an array of different landscapes, including natural environments such as forests, herbaceous borders and grasslands, compared to those typically found in urban areas such as lawns, building sites, parklands, revegetated open woodlands and remnant open woodlands. These measurements have varied greatly in locations spanning sites in the US, Canada, Australia, UK, Finland and India, but, without exception, they show that the more natural and biodiverse the environment, the more diverse and abundant the microbiota in the air, in the soil and on plant leaves.[19]

Experiments have also taken place indoors to assess what happens if we bring nature into our homes. One of my favourite and simplest examples for showing that nature's microbiota are different and better than more urban sterile environments is a study that looked at what happens to the air in a cleaned room when a spider plant (*Chlorophytum comosum*) was placed in it for six months.[20] After this time the microbial diversity of the surrounding floor and walls had a significant increase in beneficial plant bacteria (abundance and diversity). This was despite the fact that diversity on the leaves remained the same, suggesting that the plant was actively contributing to the microbial diversity in the room. Never before has the spider plant on my desk been so cherished; it is not only improving the air quality but also the microbiome on my skin and very probably the microbiome in my gut. These studies help provide a clear answer to the first assumption: more biodiverse environments have higher levels of microbial diversity – at least in the environments studied to date.

Following on from this, the second assumption that needed to be tested was that these nature-derived microbial communities are transferred and ingested into our bodies. One of the first teams to demonstrate an association between living in biodiverse environments and higher levels of microbial diversity in our bodies was led by Ilkka Hanski, of the biodiversity hypothesis fame.[21] He and his team took skin swabs from 118 teenagers living in a variety of different urban and semi-rural environments in Finland, to measure their skin microbial diversity. Clear results emerged: those who lived in environments with higher levels of biodiversity (trees, shrubs and flowering plants) had a far greater diversity and abundance of microbes on their skin. Similarly, Anirudra Parajuli and colleagues, also from the University of Helsinki, found in a study involving forty-eight elderly Finnish participants that the stool samples of those that lived in urban apartment houses with little surrounding vegetation showed much lower abundance and diversity of 'healthy' gut microbiota, compared to those in accommodation surrounded by gardens within 200 metres (220 yards) of their home.[22] However, these two studies didn't directly match the specific microbial signatures on the teenagers' skin, or the elderly people's stool samples, to those of the surrounding vegetation. So, how do we know, for example, that it is not some other feature, such as diet or pets, that is responsible for this difference (although these two studies went a long way towards excluding these aspects from influencing the result)?

Several more recent studies now appear to fill this important knowledge gap. These measured the skin and gut microbiota of the participants before and after the experiments and compared these to the environmental microbiota. The first of these studies involved participants interacting with organic soil (an important distinction because soils containing chemical fertilisers have very different and less 'good' microbiota).[23] After having their hand microbiota measured using skin swabs and genetic analysis, the participants rubbed their hands for twenty seconds in different soil and plant-based materials including composts, forest turfs, moss material and material from peat bogs: the sorts of materials we commonly encounter when gardening. They then washed their hands in water but without soap for five seconds and dried them on a paper towel. Skin swabs were then taken again for genetic analysis. What they found was a significant difference in the participants' skin microbiota after touching the soil materials. In effect, the environmental microbiome signature had transferred onto the participants' skin.

It is not hard to extrapolate from here that the environmental microbiome could also easily be inhaled and ingested – and indeed this is what was found in two other experiments. Caitlin Selway and colleagues from the University of Adelaide measured the microbiota in participants' nasal cavities (respiratory tract) before and after they had spent time in urban green spaces in Adelaide (Australia), Bournemouth (UK) and New Delhi (India), where researchers had already measured the microbial diversity in the soil, air and leaves.[24] What they showed was a clear increase in the diversity of microbiota in participants' noses and on their skin after they spent time in these biodiverse urban green spaces. Also, the microbial community composition became significantly closer to that in the air in these environments. Even though these two studies and a number of others involve only small numbers of participants and must therefore be treated as preliminary, they certainly start to suggest that when we interact in naturally biodiverse landscapes, our bodies (skin, respiratory tract and gut) adopt the microbial signature of the surrounding environment.[25]

So, assumptions one and two have been proved broadly correct: nature-derived microbiota are more abundant and diverse, and they transfer onto and into our bodies, altering our own microbiota when we are in these areas. But what about the third assumption – that this change to our microbiota triggers important changes that impact our health? Again, some tantalising findings have emerged over the last decade to suggest this is indeed the case. In the Finnish study involving teenagers, Hanski and colleagues screened their blood for specific antibodies that are known to be indicative of levels of allergies, and a strong relationship emerged.[26] Those who had the lowest levels of allergy markers in their blood lived in the more biodiverse areas. Similarly, the study involving elderly Finnish participants showed that those who lived in areas surrounded by more diverse vegetation had a reduced abundance in their gut of bacteria that are known to be pathogenic and are often used as a marker of degrading gut microbiota.[27] They also had a reduced occurrence of certain gut microbiota often associated with inflammatory bowel disease. Both these studies suggest that exposure to environmental microbiota *may* modulate our gut microbial ecology, and this *may* then influence our immune system. I say 'may' because until very recently, these studies, and similar ones, show associations rather than a direct link. Many of them also lack 'blind' controls where participants are placed in either a placebo or intervention group and the results are compared.

In the past two years, however, a series of studies have emerged to address these issues.[28] These are now starting to provide the sorts of clinically robust evidence that could, and should, be used in advising people to spend more time in nature or interacting with components enriched by it, because doing so can play an incredibly useful role in helping us to improve our immune systems.

One of the most important studies has been carried out by Maja Roslund and colleagues, again from the University of Helsinki.[29] Building on the knowledge gained in the experiment outlined at the beginning of this chapter, Roslund and her team set out to undertake what they called 'A placebo-controlled double-blinded test of the biodiversity hypothesis of immune-mediated diseases'. Even the title of this research paper sounds more clinically robust, and indeed it is. Unlike earlier studies, it involves a control (placebo) and an intervention group, and no one involved in the day-to-day delivery of the experiment knew which group they were in (hence the double-blind label).

The participants were three- to five-year-old children in kindergarten who played over a twenty-eight-day period in one of two types of sandpits for up to two hours per day. One had been enriched with a microbially diverse soil mixture, whereas the other was microbially poor with no soil. Bacterial communities in the sand, skin and stools of the children were measured before the experiment and on day 14 and day 28. Blood samples were also taken from the children before and on day 14 and the number of types of T-cells were measured. As explained earlier, T-cells are found in our blood plasma and are involved in immune function. However, depending on their type, they can play a critical role in either reducing or enhancing our auto-immune responses. In the case of the first type, the immune cells attack our own body, causing so-called autoimmune diseases. It is the balance of two different types of T-cells, called interleukin-10 and interleukin-17, that we need to worry about. Interleukin-10 (Il-10) is known to be a key player in bringing about an anti-inflammatory response – so we want as much of this in our blood as possible. On the other hand, interleukin-17 (Il-17) causes a pro-inflammatory response and is associated with diseases such as inflammatory bowel disease, rheumatoid arthritis and multiple sclerosis, so less (considerably less!) is better.

Knowing the details about these T-cells is important to appreciate the full significance of this experiment's findings. Children who played in the sandpit containing soil had a significant shift in their skin microbial diversity to become much closer in composition to the soil. And importantly their blood plasma showed a large increase in Il-10 levels (the 'good' T-cells) and a decline in Il-17. In the placebo group there was no such change in either microbial diversity or T-cell type. The children who played in the soil-enhanced sand also had higher skin microbial diversity through the duration of the experiment (day

28), suggesting that as long as the intervention is in place, the benefits will be obtained. This shows that the simple intervention of 'rewilding' the children's sandpits with microbially diverse soil had the effect of enriching their skin microbiota, associated with their immunoregulatory responses.

I find these results remarkable and extremely important. It's something so simple to do, yet potentially life-changing in terms of the long-term health benefits for the children. But adults also benefit from interacting with nature-derived microbial diversity. For example, in a recent Finnish study in which researchers looked at the effect of exposure to soil and plant materials on fourteen healthy adults, they found significance differences in their skin and gut (stool) microbial diversity.[30] During this experiment, the participants rubbed their hands with a soil- and plant-based composition three times a day for fourteen consecutive days. At the end of the two weeks not only did they show a significant increase of microbial diversity on their skin and in their guts much closer to that in the soil, but also their blood plasma had raised levels of a cytokine called TGF-β (transforming growth factor β) which is known for its ability to inhibit cell proliferation in the early stages of cancer tumours.

Suddenly, the benefits of gardening and tending our houseplants takes on a whole new dimension. As long as we are working with organically rich soils without large amounts of agrochemicals and unintentional addition of antibiotics (from cattle treated with them, for example), and not wearing gloves, then it is not just the colour, shape and smell of the plants that will be directly improving our

Richness of good skin microbial diversity in children who played in microbially diverse sandpits, compared to sterile sandpits (placebo)

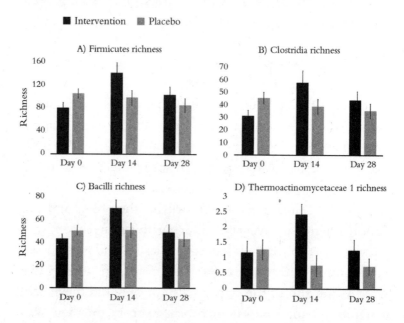

■ Intervention ■ Placebo

A) Firmicutes richness

B) Clostridia richness

C) Bacilli richness

D) Thermoactinomycetaceae 1 richness

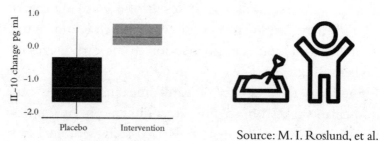

Mean change in 'good' T-cells in bloods after 28 days

Source: M. I. Roslund, et al.

health, but also the microbial diversity – a hidden sense that we obtain from the soils and plants.

This is clearly a very new and rapidly emerging field of science, and, of course, with this come large knowledge gaps yet to be filled and requiring further experimentation. Possibly one of the most important things to understand is whether interacting with nature-derived microbiota can help people who already have autoimmune and other serious diseases. Remember, the list of serious health issues that have been associated with distinctive gut microbiota is long and includes not only autoimmune diseases but also disorders such as obesity and type 2 diabetes, Alzheimer's and Parkinson's diseases, autism spectrum disorders, depression and hypertension. Yet all the experiments carried out to date have been on healthy participants. Can interacting with nature-derived microbiota and changing the gut flora of people who already have these conditions help in inhibiting and even curing some of these illnesses? Many now believe that doing so holds enormous potential for interventions of this sort but this needs to be demonstrated clinically.[31]

Another area that needs more work is the mechanism of transfer of these environmental microbes into our bodies. From the experiments described here and elsewhere we know that we inhale them, they become incorporated onto our skin and also in our gut. But what happens from this point onwards? Clearly there is strong evidence to indicate a link to changing our own microbiome to become closer to the environmental one – but why does this then trigger changes in our immune responses? It is certainly something to do with their production of secondary metabolites and other compounds and how these interact with other biochemical pathways in our bodies. But how and why this happens is still an emerging area of biomedical research.

Finally, we need to understand how long we should interact with these nature-derived microbiota to gain and maintain their benefits. Clearly short-term interaction, such as handling soil and plants, brings about changes, at least over the duration of the experiment. But do we need to do this each day to retain the benefits? A hint that we need to keep 'topping up' our environmental microbiota can be seen in the study where the Finnish participants were handling soils.[32] Although there were still differences in their microbial skin and gut diversity and blood plasma for fourteen days after the experiment, thirty-five days later these changes were no longer observed. This suggests that when we stop interacting with nature-derived microbiota, our own not-so-healthy microbiota re-establishes itself.

Having said all of this, I don't want to finish the chapter with the feeling that we need more data before we can do something. We don't. Even though the number of participants in each study is small, and many must therefore be classified as pilot studies, there are now too many of them to ignore the clear evidence emerging. When we interact with nature and its microbial diversity, this changes our own microbial diversity for the better. This change in microbial diversity can then trigger the production of secondary metabolites and other compounds with the huge potential to positively influence a plethora of autoimmune and other responses. To gain these benefits, we therefore need to be interacting with the natural environment, or aspects of it. Something as simple as a spider plant on our desk, buying and using organic soil free from inorganic fertilisers in our garden, or even having this soil contained in a cotton parcel and handling this regularly will do, as well as interacting with biodiversity outdoors. However small each of these individual actions is, what we can be certain of is that they will significantly increase the nature-derived microbiota on our skin and in our gut. And even though we can't see, hear or taste them, they will almost certainly provide us with significant health benefits – not only now, but in the long term.

8

Indoor Sensescapes: '*A garden within doores*'

How's this for a gloomy statistic: 71 per cent of all deaths globally, and rising, occur each year from non-communicable diseases, including cardiovascular conditions, heart attacks, strokes, respiratory diseases such as asthma, cancers, diabetes and mental illnesses. Even if we take into account the fact that deaths from communicable diseases, such as measles, HIV and tuberculosis, have dramatically declined over recent decades, there is still an alarming year-on-year increase in non-communicable diseases.

Also sobering is the apparently close association between increasing urbanisation and non-communicable diseases, suggesting that the two are linked in some way. This really matters, because by 2050 it is estimated that over 70 per cent of us will be living in urban environments: again a trend that is increasing year on year. The evidence for linking non-communicable diseases and other illnesses to urban environments is now so strong that it has a name: sick building syndrome.[1] It's a catch-all title for features of the built environment that make the people living and working there ill, or, at least, less well than they could and should be. Up to 30 per cent of new and remodelled buildings worldwide are now thought to be potential examples of sick building syndrome.[2]

We know that alongside urbanisation goes a large decline in the presence of nature in cities. We also know, as discussed in previous chapters, that interacting with nature through our senses can potentially result in significant physical and mental health benefits.

Sometimes global-scale problems feel too big to deal with – the worry-bucket is already overfull, and we can't take on anything else. This link between urban environments and poor health is a case in point for me. We need to live and work in urban areas, yet they seem to be killing us. Great. So, what are we supposed to do about it? Exercise more, learn relaxation techniques, improve our diet, take prescription drugs. All are well-tried and tested recommendations – but often they don't seem to move the dial in terms of death rates. Yet one recommendation that is often oddly lacking from the list, and may in fact make a significant impact, is to interact with nature more, not only outdoors, but also *indoors*. Not for the first or last time in this book, it seems that nature is the medicine.

So, can we bring nature indoors?

I believe we can, and should: indeed, we must. One of the many privileges of working in Oxford is the beauty of the physical environment that surrounds me every day. This is not just because many of the colleges and department buildings, indeed much of the city, sit gracefully in a setting of parks, courtyards, gardens, walkways and rivers. It's also because our academic ancestors brought nature inside in the form of natural materials and shapes: linen-fold panelling made of oak, chapel roof vaulting spreading like the branches of a great tree, carvings and tapestries of flowers and beasts of all kinds. My own college, St Edmund Hall, has some fine panels in our Old Dining Hall dating back to the seventeenth century. I often find myself running a surreptitious finger over their burnished surface and wondering what learned discussions and scholarly spats they have witnessed over the centuries. I find their presence comforting and conducive to concentration. Much better than the concrete breeze-blocks which form the walls of some university buildings of more recent date. Meetings held there give me a headache.

Why? What can and should we be doing about it?

This chapter sets out to understand if there are specific green design features that can capture the beneficial influence of nature even when we are indoors and reduce the negative impacts of urbanisation and sick building syndrome.

Of course, we have been incorporating nature into our indoor environments throughout the ages – both as a construction material and as a decorative feature.[3] From the earliest buildings, wood was used as a building material, because it was locally abundant and also strong and highly flexible, enabling constructions of many shapes and sizes. Structures dating from the Neolithic range from longhouses that could house up to thirty people down to small roundhouses, probably for single family dwelling, all made from wood. And even when early societies in the Near East started to use bricks and stone from around 7000 BCE, archaeological evidence suggests that wood was still used as an important construction material within these developments, as of course it still is today.

Leaping forward a few short millennia to the medieval period, you only have to glance upwards in the nave or great hall of any surviving churches or manor houses from this era to see carvings of flowers and leaves in wooden screens and panels and on stone pillars and roof bosses: wood being both used directly and imitated in stone.

Decorating the interiors of our rooms with actual houseplants and paintings and drawings of plants didn't really take off until the seventeenth century, when botany, horticulture and still-life painting of plants and other natural objects became fashionable pastimes.[4] And one book that particularly led to a surge in interest in the use of houseplants for decoration was Sir Hugh Plat's 1608 book called *Floraes Paradise*.[5]

Hugh Plat was the modern-day equivalent of a 'homes and gardens' designer. Following the success of an earlier book with the catchy title *Delights for Ladies who adorne their Persons, Tables, Closets and distillatories with Beauties, banquets, perfumes and Waters*, he had turned his hand to writing one of the first gardening manuals, *Floraes Paradise*. Particularly noteworthy is the fact that his book contained a section called 'A garden within doores', which was full of advice and opinions on the topic of indoor gardening, including details on types of plants that would work well in particular places in the home. As Catherine Horwood noted in her book *Potted History*, among other things he recommended: 'Sweet Briers, Bays and Germander' as suitable plants for shady corners of a room; advice on how to force carnations and roses to grow throughout the year; and the benefits of the resilient and long-lasting qualities of the sedum called orpin (*Hylotelephium telephium*).[6]

Many plant historians think Plat's book was the turning point for bringing plants into the home for decoration.[7] Before this time, plants were present in houses purely for medicinal and culinary purposes, at least in western Europe. Plat's book was hugely successful: it was still in print forty-two years after his death, with many later editions under the Anglicised title *The Garden of Eden*. However, the vast majority of plants recommended in Plat's book were cultivated versions of native wild plants, of the sorts found in local landscapes. All this changed from the mid-seventeenth century onwards with the arrival of 'exotick' houseplants.

As world exploration opened up ever new parts of the globe from the mid-seventeenth century, we discovered an enthusiasm for using exotic and colourful tropical blooms for indoor display. We still do. I had no idea that many of the leafy green and brightly coloured houseplants in our living rooms and workspaces (including many mentioned in previous chapters) are essentially similar to those that started to arrive in our ports and harbours around 400 years ago. Plants imported from tropical rainforests in the Americas, Africa and South-east Asia included African violets, tropical aroids (*Philodendron* spp.) and varieties with large green and shiny leaves, which can be found for sale in florists, supermarkets and garden centres today: *Anthurium, Epipremnum, Monstera, Spathiphyllum, Philodendron* and *Dieffenbachia*.[8] What I also find extraordinary is that this list would be more or less recognisable to readers pretty much anywhere in the world. I am often amazed to find that offices and homes in other countries and continents contain many of the same species of houseplants as I would find back home in the UK. We are, paradoxically, both exotic and conservative in our floral habits.

Owning exotic plants for display in homes and greenhouses was a craze throughout the Georgian and Victorian eras and into the twentieth century. 'Parlour palms' became one of the most significant decorative features in many homes, a catch-all term for varieties of palms, ferns and other hardy plants native to South America, Asia and Africa. Nor was our passion confined to the real thing: still-life paintings adorned walls and, through the work of the architects of Art Nouveau and the influence of designers such as William Morris, natural shapes began to appear in wallpaper designs, furniture and fabrics, just as they had in the carved wooden panelling and window tracery favoured by our ancestors.

However, from the late 1950s, this all changed. I think it would be fair to say that we fell out of love with nature as our choice of building material or indoors decoration. Materials such as concrete, asbestos, steel, plastic and plasterboard were in, and clean, straight-edged, functional designs became the norm. Natural materials and nature-invoked curves, shapes and patterns were no longer part of our homes, schools or offices, and plants in pots often became plastic versions. Social conditions and the rebuilding required after the devastation of war contributed too to a new sense of utilitarianism in urban design. The future was born, and it was grey. Many think this is where the demise of our physical and mental well-being in relation to our buildings began.

Fortunately, all trends bring a reaction and the 1980s saw a renewed desire to bring nature back into our indoor environments, in particular in the form of so-called biophilic design.[9]

The biologist E.O. Wilson coined the term 'biophilia' in 1984 to describe our inherent affinity for nature and our need to be surrounded by it to achieve physical and mental well-being.[10] Wilson's idea gained wide acceptance, as if he was stating something we all already knew but hadn't yet put into words. We need to conserve and surround ourselves with nature, not only for the material benefits that it can provide, but also for the positive influence it can have on our physical and mental well-being.

From here the concept of biophilic design emerged: incorporating natural features into the places where we live and work in order to enhance our connection with nature and associated well-being.[11]

This can work in three broad ways, described in a beautifully illustrated paper by Stephen R. Kellert and Elizabeth F. Calabrese in 2015. First, design using nature directly, as a feature in its own right, for example potted plants and living walls. Second, the use of indirect experiences of nature, such as pictures, natural materials and colours and the shapes and forms of nature copied in design features inside and out. Third, access to nature outside, even while inside: that is, incorporating views, sounds, natural light and open space into building design, for example in open-plan office spaces with plenty of windows.[12]

But do these indoor nature-design features have any clear health benefits? Given what we now know about smelling, seeing, hearing, touching and the hidden senses of nature described throughout the rest of the book, I would sincerely hope so! But which of these three nature design features have the most impact? And how can we apply them for maximum benefit? How many pot plants does it take to furnish a room? Does using wood as a building material really matter, given that it is often highly treated and usually brown, a colour not normally associated with promoting well-being, as noted in an earlier chapter? Are some wood types better than others? Or would it be better to paint all our walls green instead? And is more nature always better, or do we get to a point where there are too many elements of nature around us and they become a distraction?

So, taking the three elements of biophilic design in order, we start with indoor features that provide direct experiences of nature. How many potted plants should we have in a room of a given size? And what health benefits can we expect them to provide?

We know from evidence discussed in previous chapters that even a few green plants on our desks can be effective at reducing stress and providing a visual mental mini-break, and that our cognitive capabilities improve after we've looked at them. They can also improve the microbiome of the room. So, it is highly likely that even a small number of houseplants in a room will provide these benefits. But what about if we have literally hundreds of potted plants in a room, specifically in the form of an internal green 'living wall'?

Indoor green living walls are a design feature that has very much come into vogue over the past few years. In case you've never come across one – or perhaps only the outdoor versions – in essence they are vertical structures, often placed against a wall, floor to ceiling height, composed of containers of living green plants and mosses. The choice of plants is often similar to the tropical plants and ferns that we normally choose for our houseplants, as mentioned above. They are usually planted in a growing medium and have an internal watering system, so that they create a living green wall within a building. They certainly look attractive, and are found in many different sizes and shapes from small ones in individual rooms to huge expanses of living green walls in hotel lobbies, airports and other public and private buildings all over the world.

While they are most often created for their aesthetic properties, research is now starting to indicate that they could also have a significant impact on our health in three ways: by greatly ameliorating indoor air pollution, rewilding the indoor microbiome with good bacteria, and improving our mood and cognitive performance.

Let's start with indoor air pollution. My first thought was, why do we need to worry about air pollution indoors – isn't this really an outdoor problem? It seems not. Levels of air pollution indoors are typically two to five times higher than outdoors. This is because with lack of ventilation, pollutants from internal sources, such as cleaning chemicals, fabrics and building materials, become trapped and high concentrations build up in the air. Some measurements have even shown it to be as much as 100 times higher than outdoors.[13] I find that pretty alarming.

Air pollution is known to be extremely bad for our health and is responsible for a whole host of illnesses. It has been linked to increased occurrences of heart disease, lung cancer and respiratory diseases such as emphysema and asthma. It can also cause long-term damage to our nerves, brain, kidneys, liver and other organs, and it would appear that children and older people are particularly vulnerable to its impacts. Recent estimates go as far as to suggest that it is one of the greatest environmental threats to public health, globally accounting for an estimated 7 million premature deaths each year.[14] Reducing air pollution is clearly something that we should all focus on.

High levels of indoor air pollution are known to be linked to two main sources: micro-particles of dust and other organic and inorganic materials associated with furniture, carpets, construction materials and so on, and gaseous manufactured volatile organic compounds emitted from paint, varnishes and cleaning products. Plants can significantly reduce this pollution in two ways. First, they can act as an air filter owing to the tiny hairs on their leaves, which trap airborne micro-particles. Second, plants can actually absorb manufactured volatile organic compounds in their leaves via the stomata, which are the tiny openings, sometimes called pores, on the underside of leaves. The usual role of stomata is to enable gaseous exchange into and out of the plant during the process of photosynthesis; they take up carbon dioxide from the air into the leaf and give out oxygen and water. However, these stomata can also take up other compounds from the air, including for example unhealthy (for us at least) manufactured nitrous oxides, sulphur dioxide, formaldehyde, benzene and toluene.[15] When they enter the plant leaves, biochemical processes occur which helpfully break these compounds down and in effect detoxify them.[16]

So, indoor plants, particularly multiple plants situated in green walls, can potentially be an important nature-based air-cleansing system, removing both harmful micro-particles and organic volatile compounds from the air before they impact our health. But how much effect can they have? And how can we use this design feature to clear our air most effectively? Which plants, how many and where? This is where a whole new body of research is developing, including a notable study carried out by research scientists at the University of Technology in Sydney.[17] In it, they set out to test the ability of different internal living green installations in rooms to reduce indoor pollution. They chose two environments to carry out their experiments: a typical residential building in Sydney, Australia, and classrooms in Beijing, China. In the building in Sydney, three types of installation were trialled, with a fourth room as a control.

First, there was a room that contained three potted plants. The species chosen were typical houseplants: fiddleleaf fig (*Ficus lyrata*), dwarf umbrella (*Schefflera arboricola*) and 'Congo Rojo' (*Philodendron tatei*). In a second room, they placed a free-standing 1.5 square metre (sixteen square foot) vertical living green wall. This was planted with the ninety-six plants made up of species most often used for installations of this kind, including the parlour palm (*Chamaedorea elegans*), devil's ivy (*Epipremnum aureum*), fiddleleaf fig (*Ficus lyrata*), walking iris (*Neomarica gracilis*), baby rubberplant (*Peperomia obtusifolia*), peace lily (*Spathiphyllum wallisii*) and the arrowhead plant (*Syngonium podophyllum*). The third room contained a similar green wall installation to the second, but this time it had a box attached to it containing a fan designed to suck in the air from the room and funnel it up through the growing medium and over the plants before it diffused back into the room. This adaptation is known as an 'active living green wall'. Finally, in a fourth room (the control), none of these features were placed.

To quantify the amount of air pollutant removed by each intervention, the air in the rooms was first 'seeded' with a known quantity of pollutants (volatile organic compounds and micro-particles).[18] Concentrations of both in the air were continuously monitored throughout the duration of the experiment using specialised equipment to understand the effects of the different green design features.

Stark differences emerged. Even though the total duration of the experiment was short (only thirty-six minutes), the room that contained the active green wall installation, where air was sucked onto the green wall, saw a reduction of up to 75 per cent in the concentration of the volatile organic compounds and particulate matter in the air compared to the control room. The passive green wall also had lower levels of both of these pollutant types in the air compared to the control room, but this was not nearly as large a difference as was apparent with the active wall. Sadly, the three potted plants did not really make any difference: but as mentioned above, they are important for other aspects of our health – so don't ditch the aspidistra just yet!

These were empty rooms. The next question is how to make this work in a busy everyday environment. Researchers trialled the same experiment in classrooms in a school in Beijing. Once again pollution levels normally found in the ambient air were compared to those found in a classroom in which a 'free-standing' living green wall with an inbuilt plexus box was placed. Again, even over a twenty-minute period, important results emerged. In the classroom with the living green wall there was a 28 per cent reduction in volatile organic compounds and a 43 per cent reduction in micro-particles in the air. This suggests that living green walls could greatly improve air quality and provide important health benefits for children if installed in the classroom.

But what about additional benefits to children of seeing a large expanse of living green wall in the classroom? As discussed in previous chapters, children who can see green foliage from their classroom window often have improved cognitive performance.[19] So, do these interior green walls provide these additional benefits? There are still only a few studies to date that have looked specifically at indoor green walls in this way, but the emerging preliminary findings suggest that this is indeed the case, particularly with children.[20] For example, one study measured children's attentional capacity and emotional well-being in two schools in the Netherlands over a four-month period. Those in classrooms with the living green walls had much better selective attention than those in rooms with no green walls. This is important because selective attention is known to be critical to the learning process. Over time, if this trend continued, these children would perform better academically. The green wall was also shown to positively influence the children's general feelings of happiness and mental well-being associated with learning and school, which is clearly significant in itself given the gathering challenges around mental health and young people.[21]

One final thing I was curious to understand about living interior green walls was their influence on the environmental microbiome of a room. As discussed in Chapter 7, even a single spider plant was shown to positively influence the microbiome of a room. What about a whole wall full of spider plants or some other species, or a combination of different varieties of plants?

Frankly, I wasn't expecting to find any research on this, given how recent our knowledge of this topic is. Then I came across an important study carried out by scientists at the Natural Resources Institute in Finland in 2022.[22] The experiment took place over twenty days. Participants were situated in typical urban buildings. They either sat and worked in offices which had an active living green wall (the one that sucks in the air from the room and passes it over the vegetation) or no green wall (the control). Skin swabs and blood samples were taken from the participants on days 0, 14 and 28, and analysed for their bacterial diversity using genetic techniques.

What emerged should make all of us put a living green wall in our offices and workspaces. In comparison to the group that had no green wall, participants who were in the rooms with living green walls had significant changes in their skin microbiota with a much higher level of 'good' types of bacteria, known in particular to be good for skin health (*Lactobacillus*). Even more important in terms of health benefits was the finding that the participants showed a significant lowering of markers in the blood known to be associated with causing inflammation and associated inflammatory diseases. This suggests that the microbiota in their gut had changed, presumably from ingesting the microbiome in the air from the green wall, and this had triggered changes in the biochemical pathways responsible for reducing these important inflammatory markers.

Although this is only one study, evidence of this 'additional' benefit is extremely important. It suggests that such a design feature may have a significant influence on the environmental microbiome, influencing our inflammatory

Abundance of *Lactobacillus* on skin after having a green wall in office compared to no green wall

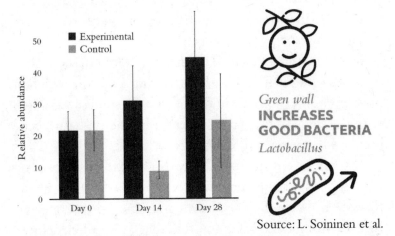

Source: L. Soininen et al.

response. Given how many non-communicable diseases are associated with enhanced inflammatory responses, this is a critically important area for further work.

The second biophilic design features are those that incorporate indirect experiences of nature, for example the use of natural materials such as wood, and a choice of colour palette that focuses on natural tones. What evidence is there that these have a positive influence on our health and well-being?

There is now a pretty substantial body of evidence to indicate that having the walls of rooms painted in natural tones, especially pastel greens, can have a calming effect. This is why so many hospital waiting rooms and corridors use these colours. But what about rooms where the walls are lined with wood? The mostly brown and patchy appearance of wood is not described as conducive to calming in any studies I have come across. Admittedly, there is evidence of calming when we *touch* wood, as discussed in Chapter 6.

But how many of us stroke the walls when we walk into a room? Yet there is clear evidence emerging from several studies that wood-lined rooms make us calmer, reduce eye fatigue and improve our cognitive performances compared to rooms finished with other materials.[23]

Why does this happen? If it is not the colour of the wood, what else might it be? Two interesting lines of evidence now emerging are hinting that it may be something to do with the smell of the wood along with other visual aspects, such as knottiness and reflectivity.

In Chapter 4, I discussed how a plant's distinctive scent comes from volatile organic compounds (VOCs) being released from the flowers, leaves and wood of the species. Also that different plants use different kinds of structures to store and release these compounds. Rosemary and lavender leaves, for example, secrete their VOCs in oil from glandular hairs on the surface of their leaves. The hairs swell like a balloon as the oils build up, releasing a scent when the leaves are touched or disturbed by the wind. Pine needles, in contrast, have resin ducts in their leaves, which are hollow tube-like structures from which the scent is emitted. Most relevant here, however, is that some species also contain vertical resin ducts not in their leaves but in their trunks.

These ducts are only found in the wood of certain families, most notably the conifers family (Pinaceae, Araucariaceae, Cupressaceae and Podocarpaceae), including many of the types that make up the majority of softwood timbers (Scots pine, European larch, Norway spruce, silver fir and Japanese cedar). Importantly, these resin ducts are not found in angiosperm tree species and in those making up hardwood timbers, such as oak, sweet chestnut and beech. The difference is very clear. Average emission values of VOCs are approximately fifty times lower from hardwood than from softwood timbers.[24]

So, the species of tree used in the panelling of the room determines the type and concentration of scent emitted into the ambient air. Even though the levels may be too low for us to notice consciously, VOCs will be present in low concentrations in the ambient air for a number of years after construction.[25] We have seen that softwoods, in particular, release terpenes (pinene and limonene), which are known to induce physiological and psychological calming. So, can we link the emission of volatile organic compounds from the types of timber used to line offices and other rooms to these health outcomes?

This question was cleverly addressed by two scientists from the Forestry and Forest Products Research Institute in Ibaraki, Japan: Eri Matsubara and Shuichi Kawai.[26] They compared participants working in a room lined with the timber of Japanese cedar (*Cryptomeria japonica*) to others working in a room with no wood cladding. Clear differences in the ambient air were detected before the experiment, with high levels of VOCs in the cedar room. In both rooms, participants took a series of thirty-minute maths stress tests specifically designed to induce anxiety. They sat behind a screen so that they couldn't see the material lining the walls of the rooms. Fascinating results emerged. Those in the unlined room showed a clear spike in their stress levels (as measured in salivary amylase) when taking the test. Those in the cedar-lined room showed no increase in stress at all. This preliminary experiment therefore hints that the volatile organic compounds emitted from certain wood types may be one of the reasons for the calming effect observed in wood-cladded rooms in previous experiments.

But what about just looking at it? Some studies are hinting that, as well as its smell, the visual qualities of certain woods can also have positive health impacts. The suggestion is that this is because typical interior wood-lining tends to have significant microscopic unevenness on the surface, associated with natural features such as knottiness. This unevenness doesn't only affect how it looks but also deflects light waves as they hit the surface. As a result, wood panels reflect only a tiny fraction of ultra-violet rays from UV lights and flickering computer screens, compared to those from surfaces made of polished and smooth manufactured materials.[27]

Some preliminary studies are starting to show that these structural features of wood as a lining material might be important for stress relief, restorativity and eye fatigue reduction. In one study, for example, participants viewed three computer graphics for ninety seconds each: two showing images of wood-lined walls composed of vertically or horizontally arranged timber and one of a simple grey image (as a control). They showed clear indications of being physiologically and psychologically calmer when looking at the images of wood. They also reported feeling 'comfortable', 'relaxed' and 'natural'.[28] In effect, looking at the wood triggered calming – similar to looking at green vegetation. Some have also suggested that natural indoor stimulation from seeing wooden interiors may be restorative because, as hypothesised in the Attention Restoration Theory (see Chapter 2), it engages our attention in a bottom-up fashion, allowing our top-down directed-attention abilities a chance to replenish.[29] In addition, the ability of wooden surfaces to reduce glare and reflectivity from computer screens and UV-B lights might also explain why working in wood-lined rooms is less fatiguing on our eyes.[30]

The benefits of wood as an indoor material might not just be confined to what's on the walls. One of the unexpected findings I came across on this topic showed that participants recovered faster from an induced stress test in an office containing oak wood furniture, compared to one with furniture made from maple wood or plastic.[31] Clearly a lot more work is needed to understand why this is the case before we all change our furniture – but it is an intriguing finding all the same.

So, emerging evidence suggests that both direct and indirect biophilic elements can be more than just design features; embedding these elements of nature in our living environments can invoke many of the same positive well-being outcomes that we get from actually being out and about in natural landscapes.

This leads me on to the third and final element of nature interior design recommended by Stephen Kellert.[32] This is where the interior design is considered as a whole 'ecosystem'. In this framing, Kellert encourages us to view space, light, views and even sounds of nature holistically, not as a series of discrete, individual elements in a room.[33,34] But what does this mean in practice? How many of these nature-inspired features do we need to find in a building to really make a difference? I would hope that more equals better, but is there a minimum number and/or are some elements more effective than others? This sort of quantitative evidence is required in order to turn these important findings into recommendations for the design of new buildings and capture their benefits in our daily lives.

Interestingly, a study to try to provide this sort of evidence at a suitably granular level of data has been recently undertaken by researchers from the Harvard Medical School, making innovative use of virtual reality (VR) headsets to create images depicting a series of different office spaces.[35,36] These VR rooms showed either tight enclosed workspaces or a more open design. In some they placed a combination of natural elements (plants and living walls), analogues of nature (pictures and photos of plants) and internal features such as wooden walls and furniture with 'natural' shapes such as a free-standing sculpture in the form of a tree. In comparison, some of the rooms had none of these features. Participants then 'visited' these office environments for five minutes each, via the VR headsets. During this time they could walk around and observe the virtual environment freely. They then sat at a desk to complete cognitive tests designed to measure reaction time and creativity. In addition, throughout the session a series of physiological measurements of levels of anxiety were taken.

Clear results emerged.[37] The participants were much calmer when visiting the open space VR rooms containing real elements of nature. Those containing natural analogues were next best. They performed worst in the closed office space with no natural elements.

Given all the evidence discussed above, I was not particularly surprised by this. However, some rather surprising findings did emerge in terms of cognitive performance. While the greatest improvement in creativity was found when the participants were in open space rooms containing natural elements, the cognitive test designed to examine reaction time (as a measure of attention) indicated the opposite: reaction time was longer in the rooms containing nature compared to the control rooms. To explain this, the authors suggested that the natural elements could be a distraction from closely attentive work. Tracking eye movements, one of the physiological measures used, certainly supports this suggestion. Participants in the rooms containing nature or their analogues spent most time looking at these features in the room.

This finding was also replicated by a team of medical scientists, architects and environmental sustainability researchers from the University of Minnesota. In their study, plants, pictures of natural scenes and recordings of birdsong were introduced into an office. Participants' levels of cognitive performance, stress, productivity and mood were measured over an eight-week period.[38] Again, subtle differences became apparent. Participants' cognitive ability to shift attention between tasks improved if they heard sounds of nature in the room while working. However, they worsened when there were too many natural elements in the room. The authors' take-home message from this study was, again, that multiple nature-design stimuli in a room may in fact become a distraction.

These preliminary results suggest that while natural elements in a room are clearly important for psychological calming, there needs to be careful consideration of what to include, taking into account the type of tasks to be undertaken in the room, and whether they are creative (such as the designers working on the jacket of this book) or attention-focused (for example the editors checking this book – they need focused attention while they work on the text in case they miss a spelling mistake!). Having said this, before we start worrying about whether having plants in our rooms will make us less productive, I do think we need to be clear about what we hope to achieve from biophilic design. If, as the increasingly large body of research is showing, it can significantly help our day-to-day levels of stress and the plethora of associated health benefits that come with this, then I believe that a little less focus in the workplace is a small price, worth paying. It may even be telling us that we need the kind of mental 'micro-break' described in earlier chapters.

The apparent ability of nature-inspired designs to make us calmer leads me on to one final recent study. A fair criticism of many of these studies is that they are looking at reactions of people who are not that stressed in the first place. Perhaps we can't therefore really determine the full impact of the designs. To address this, the team from Harvard took their use of VR headsets one step further and created a second experiment to examine whether biophilic designs in rooms can help individuals recover from a stress-induced event.[39] They hypothesised that recovery rates from stressful incidents would be faster in rooms containing natural elements, and set out to test if this was in fact the case.

A relatively large cohort of participants (100 in total) drawn from faculty, staff and students at Harvard took part. Before the experiment began, physiological stress levels were measured using the familiar tests of heart rate and heart-rate variability, skin conductance levels and blood pressure. They also filled in a questionnaire to measure their own perception of anxiety. They then took two stress-inducing tasks: a two-minute memory test and a five-minute maths test in which the questions were asked increasingly quickly, with a buzzer sounding each time an incorrect answer was given. I'd certainly find that stressful. Participants were then randomly assigned to one of four virtual reality rooms. One had no natural elements, another featured large full-length windows giving an outdoor view of green countryside, a third room contained living green walls, plants, a fish tank and wooden interiors, and finally the fourth room had both outdoor views and indoor nature features. The participants spent six minutes in their assigned room, during which their physiological and psychological parameters were continuously monitored.

The Harvard scientists found that participants in the VR room containing the natural features had consistently better recovery responses compared to those in the room with no such elements. Interestingly they also observed clear differences in the magnitude of effects between the three different types of indoor environments. The greatest physiological stress recovery occurred in the rooms with indoor natural features, but it was the room with outdoor views that had the greatest effect on the participants' perception of anxiety.

The evidence is strong and clear. Incorporating real elements of nature such as wood and plants into our homes, offices and schools will have positive benefits for both our physical and mental well-being. But, if bringing real nature inside is not practicable, all is not lost since we can still get many of these same benefits by using images, structures, sounds and colours representative of nature as an integral part of the design of our work and living spaces. And, if all else fails, viewing these features in virtual reality rooms also appears to provide some of the benefits.

Taking this line of thought one step further, we might even consider purchasing a biophilic VR headset to put on when feeling particularly stressed at work – although we might expect some rather odd looks from colleagues.

One question remained: how long do these benefits last? Most of these experiments took place over a relatively short period of time, typically up to eight weeks. Can we see longer-term impacts? Or, to put it another way, over several years, do biophilic-designed offices, homes and schools have healthier and higher performing occupants, measured over periods of years? After all, we may well spend a number of years in the same spaces in a school, home or workspace, so it's important to understand this element and get it right. As far as I am aware this is a question still requiring research, and indeed ripe for it. Biophilic design has been occurring in some buildings for over twenty years now. And we now have large, collated records of individuals' medical data available in population biobanks. The material is out there for someone to try and join it all together.

Of course, in some offices and workplaces, however, nature-inspired design is just not possible. There may not be enough room, walls may not be suitable for particular kinds of treatment, there may be nothing worth looking at outside the window, there may be nobody to water the plants or no funds to buy them in the first place. Then what? What should we do? Change jobs? Quit school?

A less dramatic option is to go for a walk at lunchtime to somewhere nearby to be immersed in nature. But, what sort of nature and for how long? This is the subject of the next chapter.

9

Outdoor Sensescapes: The Power of a Short Walk

Walking is one of the most beneficial forms of exercise. It certainly plays an important part in the routine of my own family. Weekends often involve spreading our collection of increasingly bashed Ordnance Survey maps out on the table to find an attractive new route to walk for an hour or two with our dogs, who seem to rate the enjoyment of their day by how muddy they can get and how many algae-filled duckponds they can find to leap in. Walks during the working week tend to be a bit less organised – a quick march round the park or to the bus-stop.

Both kinds are good for us. They make us feel better. And there is a strong clinical evidence base to support this. Walking doesn't damage our knee joints in the same way that jogging can do, and yet it has been shown to be associated with many of the same health benefits, including improved cardiovascular and pulmonary fitness, strengthened bones and muscles, and maintaining a healthy weight. Walking has also been associated with improved mental well-being.

But I think it is fair to say that not all walks are equal in terms of health benefits.

Broadly speaking walks fall into two categories. First, there is walking as a planned leisure activity, in countryside near our homes or on a more structured and energetic hike further afield. The health benefits of this kind of walk are easy enough to understand. Second, there is walking as a component of doing something else, such as getting to school or work or nipping to the shops. Most of these kinds of walks are in a town or city. They usually come with noise, traffic, pollution and other distractions attached, and they are rarely a leisurely stroll but rather a dash to get from point A to point B for a meeting, to catch the shop before it closes, or even to fit in a quick phone call.

It is with the second category, walking in cities and urban areas, that the health benefits become less clear. Even though walking (and jogging) in these environments will still be good for certain aspects of our health such as strengthened bones and muscles, they can also have a negative impact on our pulmonary fitness (think respiratory illnesses associated with pollution), anxiety levels (think cardiovascular illnesses associated with stress) and mental well-being. Walking in cities can be detrimental to our health.

So far, this book has presented plenty of evidence that interacting with nature offers health benefits simply by seeing, hearing and smelling the natural environment. The obvious inference, therefore, is that we ought to be able to mitigate some of the nasty aspects of walking in an urban environment simply by taking a slightly longer, less direct route that takes in as much nature as possible. But what sorts of nature, and for how long?

In cities there are several types of green infrastructures that we might easily be able to encounter with a bit of route planning. Broadly, we can group these under three headings: fully green-space urban parks, urban streets with trees, and smaller introduced features such as planters, window-boxes and vertical external green walls. What benefits do they provide? And for how long do we need to be encountering them to gain these benefits? This chapter will look at these three different aspects of urban greenery.

Starting with the benefits of taking a brief lunchtime stroll in the nearest park rather than on the streets, the scientific evidence gives us clear instructions: head for the park. Walking in the park compared to the streets will make us physiologically and psychologically calmer even if travelling at the same speed and in the same weather conditions. With this comes a whole host of other health benefits.[1] One of my favourite examples demonstrating these benefits was an experiment led by Professor Chorong Song, from the University of Chiba.[2]

This took place in Kashiwa city in Japan and involved male participants, all of similar age (about twenty-two years old), height, weight and health, taking a pre-determined route for fifteen minutes either in a large urban park containing many hardwood trees such as maple, tulip, cherry and chestnut, or on streets in a nearby area. Some walked the city route first and then the park, and others vice versa. They all maintained similar average walking speeds throughout, and no alcohol or tobacco consumption was allowed during the experiment. The weather was also the same on the three days when the experiment took place; so, as far as possible, the individuals and their activities were comparable throughout. During the walks, the participants wore a portable electrocardiograph to measure their heart rate, and after each walk, they filled in two questionnaires, designed to measure their mood and anxiety levels.

Even though this was a relatively simple study, clear differences were found in all measures. The participants were much calmer and exhibited significantly lower levels of negative emotions and anxiety when walking in the urban park compared to the streets.

I was not entirely surprised by this finding – and if you've come this far with me in this book, I hope you won't be either. From the evidence I have reviewed so far I would be confident in inferring that the physiological and psychological calming found in the participants is almost certainly something to do with their interaction with the colours, shapes, smells and sounds of nature in the park. Another promising avenue of research is related to our propensity to ruminate less when walking in nature. Rumination is one of those words that has two totally different meanings. To quote one dictionary:

- a deep or considered thought about something; 'philosophical ruminations about life and humanity'.
- the action of chewing the cud

We can leave the second to the cows, but the first has been the focus of some interesting research to understand what we think about when walking in city spaces with trees compared to treeless areas. This is of particular interest because introspective thought can become negative and destructive, leading to negative thoughts about oneself, or worse. This type of rumination is often associated with a raised risk of depression and other mental illnesses. Some mechanisms that distract from rumination are themselves harmful, such as binge drinking. A much better option is nature acting as a distraction. So, can this work on our urban walk?

Gregory Bratman and colleagues from Stanford University set about to address this question by randomly assigning participants who all lived in urban areas and with no history of mental illness to carry out a ninety-minute walk. These were either in a green space with scattered oak trees and shrubs near to the university, or on a street in Palo Alto with four lanes of traffic and a constant flow of vehicles.[3] Before undertaking the walk, the participants filled in the Reflection Rumination Questionnaire. In addition, they underwent brain imaging in order to detect the volume of blood flowing to the part of the brain called the subgenual prefrontal cortex. Blood flow to this area has been shown to increase during times of sadness and rumination. The same tests were then carried out on their return.

Clear findings emerged: those participants that went on the ninety-minute walk in the park showed significant reductions in self-reported rumination and decreases in brain activity in the subgenual prefrontal cortex, whereas those who went on an urban walk did not show these effects.

Given the documented link between rumination and the risk of depression and other psychological illnesses, Bratman and his colleagues concluded that the reduction in rumination among those walking in the park with trees is one possible mechanism by which urbanisation and its associated loss of nature experience may be linked to mental illness. Therefore, at a neurobiological level, a walk in city areas with trees and other aspects of nature may be one action that provides us with an additional important benefit to protect against mental illness.[4]

Which leads me on to my next question. Are there some parts of the park or styles of landscaping that are better to walk in than others? As discussed in previous chapters, many of the benefits of interacting with nature are associated with different senses. We also know that the spatial distribution of nature is not homogenous and that, as discussed in Chapter 1, there are some outlines of landscapes that have better health outcomes when we view them than others. The question is, then, how does this translate into our urban landscapes and in particular the designs of parks that we have in our cities?

The term urban park was first coined in the seventeenth century. Over time they became associated with a desire to enable the working poor to access green space in cities for exercise and contemplation, as the industrial revolution had increasingly brought work and working people into cities where such opportunities were limited.[5]

In the UK, some of the first urban parks were created from 1833 onwards in cities typically associated with ironworks and cotton mills. Many were funded by public subscription. As part of the deal, subscribers were able to purchase land to build houses overlooking the park – an option that worked well.[6] Many of these large Victorian and Edwardian houses can still be seen standing elegantly alongside urban parks in both the UK and many western European cities, and they remain extremely desirable (and often very expensive) places to live. People like being close to nature, and will pay for the privilege.

Another legacy that is still apparent is the structure and form of these public gardens. According to the prevailing tastes of the day, these urban parks were designed in formal geometric patterns with highly ordered colourful herbaceous borders interspersed with neatly manicured lawns. Sometimes they included features such as lakes, tennis courts and spaces for musical events such as bandstands. Again, many of these additional features still exist in parks in the UK and elsewhere. Their overarching ethos is one of regularity, order, and nature organised and controlled. In many ways, they recreate the sense of balance and decorum of a classical or renaissance garden.

It should be noted here, however, that other notable campaigners took a rather different approach, focused on preserving large, wooded wilderness-type areas on the edges of cities. Octavia Hill (1838–1912), for example, successfully campaigned to save both Hampstead Heath and Parliament Hill Fields in north London from development; both are now seen as iconic green spaces in London. It was Hill who first used the term 'green belt', and she was a major player in improving housing for the urban poor and their access to open spaces for 'the life-enhancing virtues of pure earth, clean air and blue sky', as she aptly put it. She also co-founded the National Trust with Canon Hardwicke Rawnsley and Sir Robert Hunter, with significant early contributions from naturalists such as the children's author Beatrix Potter, again inspired by concern about protecting and preserving open spaces for everyone to access.

The first urban parks in the US were more aligned with the wilderness model, no doubt partly at least because America's big cities have emerged much more recently and often in places with much more space around them, rather than developing organically on the small footprint of an industrial, medieval or even Roman settlement in a geographically confined location, as is so often the case in the UK and other parts of Europe.[7] American parks were created in response to similar problems – the need to provide spaces in cities for relaxation, contemplation and recreation for the working poor. Their style was aligned with the early philosophical writings of the pioneering American naturalists Ralph Waldo Emerson and Henry David Thoreau. They believed that nature would only give us full respite and stimulate and exercise the unused part of the mind if we allow ourselves to attune to its wilder aspects. The idea here, therefore, was that urban parks should be seen as 'pieces of the country with fresh air, meadows and lakes', but right in the middle of the city.

This concept was enthusiastically embraced by early urban landscape gardeners in the US, notably Frederick Law Olmsted, who from 1858 designed Central Park in New York City and the Golden Gate Bridge Park in San Francisco, among others. He aimed to create a wilderness atmosphere with romantic, irregular clusters of shrubbery, interspersed with patches of open ground and winding paths. Little attention was given to colourful flower beds or geometric shapes, although there were areas for sports such as baseball and ice skating, and spaces for making and listening to music. Both these parks still have this character today: they are very different from London's Regent's Park or Victoria Park, for example.

Interestingly, both models have spread and found favour away from the places where they were originally created. Many European cities have parks that attempt to emulate the US-style focus on the wilder type of park, but the US itself also boasts more formal European-style gardens, such as the famous Huntington Botanical Gardens in California, laid out in 1919. Today, examples of both types can be found in and around most large cities across the world.

So, what sort of design of urban park is better for walking in? Is it the design with its less formal structure and a nod to wilderness, or it is the neat and ordered version with areas of grass interspersed with flowerbeds, of the beneficial sort mention in Chapter 2, originating from our tidy-minded Victorian ancestors?

Well: it depends. For example, if we are looking for physiological calming from viewing the landscape then research shows that wilder urban gardens can provide more relaxation. At least these were the findings of a study devised by researchers from the National College of Natural Medicine, Portland, Oregon, in the western US. They measured physiological and psychological changes in participants when they walked for twenty minutes in four different areas of urban 'naturalness': two urban parks (wild and ordered), a tree-lined street and a highly urbanised street.[8] What they found was that the wild urban park containing scattered trees, shrubs and other natural elements with minimal evidence of human influence, provided the greatest pre-to-post change in stress. The next best stress-buster was the urban park with walkways and other built recreation features. Third came the street where the majority of viewable landscape is due to human influence, with some natural elements such as trees. The least calming was the walk in densely built areas where almost everything in sight was human-created.

Another benefit of the more wild types of urban gardens could be from birdsong. We know that hearing songbirds can lead to physiological calming and, generally, it is likely that the wilder the landscape, the more birds there are.[9] This is because these landscapes will potentially provide greater habitats for nesting and foraging. Also, small songbirds tend not to be found in large open spaces, such as the expanses of open grassland which are typical of some urban parks, because of the risks of predation. So to hear birdsong in the city we need to seek out wilder areas and stay close to small hedges and trees (and remove our headphones).

However, we do need to be careful not to assume that all wilderness-style urban parks are always better at relieving stress for all users. I say this because evidence also suggests that too many trees and shrubs can in fact have the opposite effect and actually raise levels of stress. For example, Birgitta Gatersleben and Matthew Andrews from the University of Surrey carried out a study in which participants were shown photos of an urban park with a successively greater density of wooded areas in each photo.[10] They found that there was an increased amount of physiological and psychological stress as the areas became more wooded. To then determine whether these emotion responses had a measurable impact in a real-world situation, a second experiment was carried out in which participants took two walks, one in an environment with a high density of trees and little view, the other having a more open landscape with fewer trees. Again, clear differences emerged: when walking in the environments with a view and relatively few trees, the participants' heart rates were significantly lower, and their mood and attention was better compared to when they walked in an area that was predominantly wooded.

Why this occurs is thought to be due to the environmental psychological theory of 'prospect and refuge', which was first proposed by John Appleton in 1975.[11] This sought to explain why certain environments feel secure when we are in them. Appleton suggested that people feel safer in environments that provide the capacity to observe (prospect) without being seen (refuge for example from potential attack), so we prefer environments with high prospect and high refuge.

However, others have since challenged Appleton's hypothesis, pointing out that while environments with high refuge can be a good place for a potential victim to hide, they can be a place for potential attackers to hide as well. This was the starting point for the study carried out by Gatersleben and Andrews referred to above.[12] So, their findings are significant, because they show a different outcome from Appleton. Individuals feel less stressed and find landscapes most restorative, at least in the urban country parks used in this experiment, where there are high levels of prospect, and *low* levels of refuge (i.e. fewer places for attackers to hide). I think most urban dwellers, especially women, would relate to this finding. I certainly do; dark leafy areas of urban parks make me feel stressed, and I try to avoid them. City planners take note: seeing too many trees in an urban park is not necessarily restorative.

When it comes to viewing more formal-style gardens, we must also remember that there are benefits to be had from seeing their colourful flowering borders. As discussed in Chapter 3, a number of studies demonstrate that when we view flowerbeds with greater colour and diversity of flowers we have greater levels of happiness and stress recovery.[13]

But for me, one of the most important benefits that we obtain from these herbaceous borders is from their smell (see Chapter 4). Many contain lavender, rosemary, mint, roses and other plants that emit volatile organic compounds known to trigger significantly positive physiological and psychological changes in our bodies. And, after researching the potential effects of volatile organic compounds on our health for this book, I have become a total convert. I think smell is one of the most beneficial and yet under-researched aspects of nature's way of keeping us healthy. By smelling certain plant compounds we can enhance our immune system and reduce inflammation and allergic responses.[14]

Remember – it is not a plant's scent that causes hay fever; it is the pollen grains. This distinction often gets muddled (perhaps understandably, since both get up our noses). On the whole plant smells are very good for us. I therefore find it puzzling how little we acknowledge the importance of plant scents in urban parks, wild or ordered. And when areas with good scents are identified, they are usually badged as a sensory garden for those with disabilities – as if they are only of interest and importance to those who do not have the benefit of the other senses. Smell is almost a forgotten sense. In future, if we are serious about gaining the maximum health benefit from nature in these urban parks, then along with maps detailing where to find the most colourful herbaceous borders, we ought to have smellscape maps, detailing where and in which months we should seek out and experience these various smells. Even now, the advice to walk in areas of the park that contain coniferous trees including cedar, cypress and pine trees or scented herbaceous plants in summer months would be a start, since we already know that these trees release many important volatile organic compounds associated with specific health benefits.

Both wilder and more ordered urban parks therefore offer benefits from seeing, hearing and smelling nature. But what about hidden senses in the environmental microbiome? Some of the early experiments looking at our skin and gut microbiota clearly showed that different urban areas have distinctive microbial differences, including the finding that areas with greater levels of biodiversity have a more diverse and beneficial microbiome. But can this finding be translated into how we design and use urban parks? And what types of parks are best in this respect?

Although there is relatively little research on this so far, a recent study carried out in an urban park in Adelaide, Australia, suggests that to interact with a biodiverse environmental microbiome we should head for the wilder parts of the park and avoid the open grassy areas. In this 2021 pilot study, three habitat types were measured: grasslands, bare soil and scrub habitats containing eucalyptus trees and bushes.[15] A particularly novel aspect of this experiment was the fact that vertical stratification of the environmental microbiome was measured. This was achieved by constructing a wooden framework on which petri dishes containing agar gel, which captures bacteria on its surface, were fixed at heights of 0.5 metres, 2 metres and 5 metres (1.6 feet, 6.5 feet and 16.4 feet) – the former two equate to a child in a pushchair and a tall adult – in order to capture the bacterial communities. In this way, the environmental biota could be measured both at ground level and at these levels above the vegetation. Understanding this vertical stratification is important because the closer the bacterial loads are to our skin and respiratory tract, the more likely we are to ingest them, and they then become part of the microbiome in our gut.

What emerged from this study were large differences in the composition of the microbiota of the different habitats, both in type and also in how high off the ground they were. The most diverse and vertically stratified communities were found in areas with scrub habitats containing eucalyptus trees. A strong linear relationship was also found between a higher density of trees and closer tree canopies in these areas and a higher microbial diversity. In contrast, the areas with the lowest levels of microbiota were found in areas of grassland. In fact, the grasslands did not fare at all well. They were found to contain a larger number of the types of bacteria that can cause disease (identifiable pathogenic species) compared to the samples from the scrub habitats, which contained a high abundance and diversity of 'good' bacteria. There was also little vertical stratification of the microbiota in the air above the grasslands (although if these are the pathogenic bacteria, then this is probably not such a bad thing after all).

So, in addition to my comments about the need to create 'smellscape' maps of urban parks, this pilot study suggests that we also need to consider creating maps showing areas containing high concentrations of good environmental biota. Or, to flip it around, we should be working out ways to enhance the environmental biota in urban parks. Although this might sound a bit far-fetched, some have already suggested this in the microbiome rewilding hypothesis.[16] This proposes that if we restore biodiverse habitats in urban green spaces we will rewild the environmental microbiome, and this will enhance primary prevention of human disease. A pretty strong claim – but something I think we need to take extremely seriously, especially given the potential health benefits from interacting with the environmental microbiome as outlined in Chapter 8.

But is this possible? Jacob Mills and his colleagues from the University of Adelaide, who proposed this hypothesis, certainly think so. In evidence they point to studies of former landscapes that have been rewilded with native vegetation, showing that the microbiome in the soil community followed suit. The microbiome was more diverse and abundant in as little as eight years.

So, it would appear that both wilder and more formal urban green spaces offer benefits by triggering reactions through our senses when we walk in them. It would be good to think that city planners and urban landscape architects actively consider this aspect when designing green spaces in our towns and cities, as well as important other factors such as air quality, space for recreation and social interaction, and wildlife connectivity.

Another critical question is: how long should we walk in these urban parks for? Will a quick ten-minute trot around the park once a week be OK – or do we need to spend longer than this? If so, how long, and how often? A couple of recent studies have come up with some startlingly clear recommendations: we should walk in nature for at least twenty minutes at a time, and spend at least 120 minutes per week immersed in nature to gain its full benefits for health and well-being.[17]

This twenty-minute figure emerged from a neat study designed by Mary Carol Hunter and colleagues at the University of Michigan.[18] They set up an experiment to determine how much stress relief was gained by taking walks of differing lengths in natural settings. Participants, who were faculty and staff at the university and of a similar age (about fifty years old), were asked to undertake a nature experience (sitting, walking or a mixture of both) three times a week over an eight-week period. The study was designed to emulate 'real life' as closely as possible, so that during the eight-week period, the participants chose when to take the walk and how long to walk for (as long as it was during daylight hours and longer than ten minutes). To measure the reduction in stress associated with these different lengths of walks, the participants took salivary swabs before and after their walks so that cortisol and salivary amylase could be measured in their samples. As noted earlier, both are known to be good clinical measures of stress. Intriguing results emerged. While the participants' lengths of walks were reasonably well distributed across four different lengths of time (seven to fourteen minutes; fifteen to twenty minutes; twenty-one to thirty minutes and more than thirty minutes), distinctive differences emerged in the cortisol and salivary amylase values associated with these times. Somewhat counter-intuitively, the optimal time to spend in nature was between twenty and thirty minutes. Shorter than this and the evidence for stress reduction was significantly smaller, more time than this and even although the benefits continued to accrue, this was at a greatly reduced rate.

Another interesting finding was that the greatest drop in salivary amylase, indicating a reduction in stress, occurred while the participants were sitting, or with a combination of sitting and walking. Their stress relief was considerably better, in fact, than if they were just walking or running. Given that this is a single study, these results should only be treated as preliminary, and I certainly don't want to irritate all those who enjoy running by saying that they would get better stress relief if they stopped and sat down – running has a whole host of other health benefits that also need to be taken into consideration. All the same, it is potentially good news for those of us who do occasionally feel the need for a bit of a sit-down when out on a run or country ramble. It suggests that anyone can get health benefits from just being immersed in nature – as long as we do it for at least twenty minutes. This preliminary finding also very much aligns with the large body of research that is emerging on the practice of forest bathing.[19] It would appear that 'park bathing' in cities can provide similar benefits.

So, if twenty minutes is the right duration for each visit, how many times each week should we be doing this? The study that came up with the '120 minutes a week' suggestion was led by Matthew White and colleagues at the University of Exeter.[20] They cleverly made use of a very large dataset from a UK survey called 'Monitor of Engagement with the Natural Environment Survey' (MENE). This is an annual exercise carried out as part of the UK government's collation of national statistics and involves around 4,000 people being surveyed each week across England for fifty-two weeks of the year. Among many other things, they are asked about how often and how long they have spent in the natural environment in the preceding seven days. They are also asked questions relating to their self-reported health (good versus poor) and subjective well-being (high versus low). Data from the years 2014–16 involving survey responses of around 20,260 people allowed White and his team to compare the health and well-being responses of these individuals with the frequency and duration of reported time they spent each week in nature (rounded to sixty-minute blocks). What they found was that the likelihood of people reporting 'good health' and 'high well-being' was significantly higher when they spent 120 minutes or more in nature during the week. Less than this showed no relationship. These positive associations continued and peaked at 200–300 minutes, indicating that more is better, but only up to this point – beyond this, little further benefit is gained.

What I also found interesting from this study was that it didn't appear to matter if this nature experience was taken as one large block or lots of smaller walks, and that this pattern was consistent across all age and health groups, including older people and those with long-term health issues. Even for people who live in areas with very little green space nearby, this more than 120 minutes threshold was apparent, presumably meaning that these participants travelled for their green space fix.

Now, moving on to the final two features of nature that we sometimes encounter in cities: street trees and vertical living green walls. What health benefits, if any, do they confer?

Street trees have been planted in cities since the earliest civilisations, with clear evidence for formal protection of them dating as far back as 1755 BCE.[21] The Babylonian Hammurabi code, the longest, best-organised and best-preserved legal text from the ancient Near East refers to a number of accepted codes of practice and prohibitions, including one on not cutting down trees. Not for the first time in researching this topic, I was confronted with how clearly our ancestors understood the importance of nature.

The beneficial use of street trees is well documented, covering many aspects ranging from sustainable street furniture and green design features to nature-based environmental solutions for providing shade, reducing the urban heat-island effect and controlling pollution.[22] The world over, a relatively small selection of tree species are used for street planting. These tend to be chosen because of the pretty shape of their foliage (e.g. maidenhair trees, *Ginkgo biloba*), their ability to withstand pollution (e.g. plane trees, *Platanus* x *acerifolia*), their resistance to heat and wind (e.g. callery pear, *Pyrus calleryana*), or some other feature such as their autumn leaf colours (e.g. American sweet gum, *Liquidambar styraciflua*) or sweet fragrances in midsummer (e.g. *Tilia cordata*, small-leaved lime).

Some street trees, however, do offer problems for urban planners, and these can include those which produce a sticky sap that adheres to car windows, tree roots that protrude through the pavements and undermine walls and surfaces, and, in some species, highly allergenic pollen. In terms of pollution control, we also have to be careful not to overplay the role of street trees because in the wrong place, such as the central reservation, they can sometimes have the opposite effect and reduce street ventilation by trapping and acting as a concentration for pollutants (the so-called canyon effect).

The suggestion that more street trees will reduce respiratory diseases, and in particular childhood asthma, must also be treated with caution since some trees can trigger allergic responses. Indeed, a recent systematic review to assess current evidence upended the oft-cited statement that 'more street trees result in lower incidences of childhood asthma': many studies do not find this association.[23] Surprising though it may seem, it seems there is currently no scientific consensus that urban trees reduce asthma by improving air quality. It's all about putting the right number of the right trees in the right places.

This is a bit of a health warning against reaching too readily for what looks like the obvious conclusion. But at the same time, we have to be careful not to just concentrate on respiratory health in relation to street trees because there are many studies emerging showing highly positive associations between them and other aspects of health. Several large population-scale studies show significantly lower levels of cardiovascular diseases and mental illness in areas with a higher abundance of street trees, including for example the fine lakeside city of Toronto in Canada.[24]

This city has many things to recommend it but of most relevance here is its knowledge of its street trees. The Toronto Street Trees Data Set lists the location and species type of over 530,000 individual trees growing on public land in the city. Toronto also has an excellent dataset on individuals' health and demographics called the Ontario Health Study which contains the health records of 31,109 people. A study carried out at the University of Chicago used these two datasets to compare the number of trees on a street with health outcomes for the people who lived there, with some clear findings emerging.[25] There was a positive association between cardiovascular health and tree density, meaning that those who lived in areas where there was a greater number of trees on a sidewalk had a lower incidence of cardio-metabolic conditions. They also felt better about their health and general well-being. These results remained statistically strong even when controlling for other socio-economic and demographic factors.

Around the same time as this paper was published in 2015, another study appeared, this time looking at mental health and street trees in London. A similarly positive correlation emerged. Researchers investigated whether there was any association between urban street tree density and antidepressant prescription rates.[26] London is divided administratively into thirty-three boroughs, and for each of these there is publicly available data from the UK National Health Service that details the number of prescriptions given each year for antidepressants. There is also data for each London borough on the location and number of trees, enabling a calculation of the density of trees on pavements in each street. After accounting for other factors such as unemployment levels, mean age of population in each borough and percentage of smokers, there was still a strong inverse association apparent; that is, London boroughs with a higher density of trees on the pavements had statistically lower rates of prescribing for antidepressants.

Searching the literature suggests that these studies are not just 'one-offs' and peculiar to these specific cities. A number of similar studies have replicated these findings from other cities all across the world, suggesting that people who live and walk in areas with more street trees have reduced incidences of cardiovascular illnesses and better mental health.[27]

But how does this work? What these studies are showing is an association between health outcomes and number of trees – but usually not the changes in our bodies that lead to these improved health outcomes. Taking into account the large body of evidence discussed throughout this book indicating that sensing nature around us triggers a whole host of physiological and psychological health benefits, I think it would be fair to say that these associations are probably due to a mixture of these interactions – but which ones, and for how long we need to be living and walking on these streets, is still unclear. This is definitely an area that warrants further research. More studies like the ones mentioned at the beginning of this chapter, comparing park to street walking, would be a good place to start. For example, if you walk in streets with trees compared to those without, what are the physiological and psychological differences that occur in your body? To my knowledge this sort of detailed experiment has yet to be done, but it needs to become a high research priority.

Having said this, I did come across a really interesting study which examined whether there is a link between the number of trees and shrubs around people's homes (the study looked for vegetation greater than 0.7 metres, about 30 inches in height), and levels of depression, anxiety and stress. In this study researcher Daniel Cox and colleagues asked: if you increase the percentage of tree and shrub cover around an individual's home, is there a corresponding reduction in stress, and if so, by how much? The study was carried out in an urban area in southern England known as the Cranfield Triangle, which covers the three adjacent towns of Milton Keynes, Luton and Bedford. Self-reported measures of mental health (levels of depression, anxiety and stress) were obtained from 263 participants living in the Cranfield Triangle, and the individuals' results were compared to percentage cover of trees and shrubs more than 0.7 metres (about 30 inches) in height around a 250-metre (275-yard) radius of their homes.

Clear findings emerged. Even when taking other variables such as poverty and income into account, the odds of suffering from depression, anxiety and stress were significantly lower when at least 20–35 per cent of the landcover around an individual's house was trees and shrubs.

Using this data, Cox and his colleagues estimated that if all the participants lived in neighbourhoods with around 20 per cent of the vegetation cover being trees and shrubs, the total number of symptoms of depression, anxiety and stress in the Cranfield Triangle could be reduced by up to a quarter. They also estimated that this could bring about a national annual saving of between £0.5 and £2.6 billion a year on health bills for depression.[28] This is a pretty astonishing finding, and definitely the sort of saving that makes policy makers, who can be quite dismissive of nature's value in cities, start to listen. Trees save money by making us less sick. What politician or planner would turn their back on that double whammy of wins?

The final type of urban nature infrastructure I wanted to understand in terms of its health benefits includes the kind that seem to be springing up all over the world: green walls. As mentioned in earlier chapters, these are plants grown on a vertical wall, and they come in two main types: either the plants are climbers, rooted in soil at the bottom and trained to grow up a trellis, or the plants are grown in planter boxes, which are then slotted onto a frame attached to the wall. Both are commonly referred to under the term vertical green walls. Even though in some cities these might still seem like a local design feature, the number of green walls in cities and the spaces they cover is rapidly increasing globally. Singapore is currently top of the green-wall leader board with a target, likely to be met, of 80 per cent of its buildings to be covered in green walls by 2030. But the world's largest single expanse of a green wall is in Khalifa Avenue in Qatar, covering 7,000 square metres (8,380 square feet), while the tallest green wall grows 92 metres (100 yards) up the side of a residential building in Medellín in Colombia.

Even though vertical green walls might seem a recent invention, in fact they originated in the US in the 1930s. The first vertical green-wall system was developed by a professor of Landscape Architecture at the University of Illinois called Stanley Hart White. He created prototypes in his back garden in Illinois which he called 'botanical bricks'. Some prefer to claim, however, that the first vertical green wall designs date back much earlier to ancient Babylon (today's Iraq), where legend suggests that around 600 BCE King Nebuchadnezzar II built a large hanging garden, with plants interwoven into brick terraces, to offer solace and succour to his wife because she was missing the abundant plants and associated wildlife from her home country. Perhaps these were the first real vertical green walls. In any case, it's always nice to introduce a dash of romance, so let's go with it.

Choice of plants in these green walls is strongly dependent on whether the structure has an internal watering system, and the local climate. An installation with an internal watering system in place, set in a warm and temperate climate, may well feature flowering native plants, hardy tropical houseplants and bromeliads. If, however, the feature does not have an internal watering system and/ or the installation is in a harsher climate, the plants will naturally be those known to be resistant to drought, frost and heat, including for example hardy grasses, ivy, ferns, succulents and mosses.

Vertical green walls are often placed in areas in cities where there is simply not enough space for horizontal green expanses – by definition, the most built-up parts. And many major cities across the world are sprouting vertical green walls; every time I visit London these days I seem to spot another one. As mentioned above, however, the capital city for vertical green walls has to be Singapore. Singapore is often called the Garden City because of the incredible amount of green foliage covering the walls of even some of its most high-rise buildings. It has seen a surge in these types of installations since 2009 when strong government support and financial incentives led to the greening of many iconic high-rise buildings. I think it would be fair to say, however, that research into the benefits associated with vertical green walls has, until recently, been predominantly focused on their role in greenhouse gas removal and air pollution reduction.[29] There is now strong evidence to indicate that they can be very good at this and can significantly lower levels of particulate matter in the air around them, with the interesting finding that the greater the biodiversity of plants, the more particulate matter they seem to trap.[30]

But in addition to pollution removal, do green walls confer any other health benefits? The few studies that have addressed this question to date are revealing some really interesting findings.[31] They suggest that viewing vertical green walls can trigger the same sort of physiological and psychological calming as viewing green horizons (Chapter 2). For example, when Mohamed Elsadek and colleagues from Tongi University in China compared results from brain activity, heart-rate variability, skin conductance and questionnaires recording mood and levels of anxiety of a group of participants who looked at a vertical green wall at a 1.5-metre (five-foot) distance for five minutes, and compared these to when they spent a similar time looking at a simple brick wall, very clear differences emerged.[32] All of these parameters clearly indicated physiological and psychological calming when looking at the vertical green wall, which was not present when viewing the bricks.

Clearly more studies are needed to understand this relationship better, not least how much the choices of what we plant in them affects these outcomes, and what other benefits green walls might provide, for example enhancing the environmental microbiome. But even these preliminary results offer cause for hope and encouragement. They

234

suggest that, as our cities become more built up, vertical greening may well still provide some of the benefits that we would otherwise gain from seeing biodiverse green space at ground level. Just as town planners in the 1950s and 1960s decided to turn the idea of the urban residential street through 90 degrees and stand it on its end to poke up into the sky (with mixed results), so we should now learn to do the same with our urban gardens.

The studies discussed in this chapter and the last have left me feeling a lot more positive about living in an urban environment. They suggest that we don't have to fall victim to non-communicable diseases or less good mental health because we live in cities. We can use and benefit from nature around us, indoors and outdoors, to reduce some of the worst effects of urbanisation. But to do so, we need to think more consciously of nature as something that we should routinely interact with in our everyday activities, even, perhaps especially, in our daily dash between our important and competing activities, and not as a discrete 'nice to have' that we fit in when we have time and aren't too exhausted (or, more often, don't).

We also now have enough data to give us a pretty good idea of which aspects of nature we should try and incorporate in our everyday walks, and for how long each week. If finding these different elements all sounds a bit too much like hard work, then be reassured that many of the good smells, sights, sounds and hidden senses of nature tend to overlap and are found in areas with more diverse vegetation. This is what we should search out. Walking around a flat area of grass such as a football pitch will simply not provide these benefits. And anyway, it's boring.

If you instinctively like the sight, sound or smell of where you are walking, it is probably doing you good. Make time to do more. Walk to work, at least some of the way. Walk with your children to school, and find the most nature-intensive route you can. You will be embedding good learning, good health and good habits for life.

10
Digging for Health

No book on green senses would be complete without talking about gardening. It's a hugely popular pastime for many of us: around 42 per cent of the UK population currently classify themselves as gardeners. Similarly, around 55 per cent of American households engage in gardening activities, which translates to 71.5 million gardening households. Another way of judging our global attraction to gardening is to look at how much we spend on it. Again, the figures are surprisingly large. In 2020, for example, the global garden care market was around $104 billion (£82 billion), and this is increasing annually.[1] As a comparison, the annual worldwide market in golf equipment and apparel is estimated at around $20–25 billion (£16–20 billion).

Interestingly, however, there are also large cultural differences in our propensity to garden.

An online global survey in 2017, which asked 23,000 consumers from seventeen countries 'how often do you garden?' revealed clear distinctions.[2] Apparently, Australia has the highest percentage of daily or weekly gardeners, followed by China, Mexico, the US and Germany. In contrast, South Koreans are the least likely to garden, with more than half of the respondents to the survey indicating they had never taken part in this activity. Other countries with high percentages of 'never-gardened' responses included Japan, Spain, Russia and Argentina. It is worth noting, however, that these figures have probably changed since the 2017 study, following the Covid pandemic. Numerous studies from across the world indicate that people took up gardening during Covid. For example, in the UK, over seven million people started gardening during the first lockdown, and this number has not declined since.

Why do we garden? To the uninitiated, the idea of grubbing about in the soil getting mud under fingernails and inadvertently touching a worm might seem unhygienic, and a good reason not to do it. Yet when 6,000 people in the UK were asked this question, the prime motivator they gave was for the pleasure that gardening brought them.[3] Similar responses have been found in many other regions in the world. It would appear that we garden because we enjoy it, the same as any other outdoor hobby.

We don't, it seems, consciously choose gardening specifically for its health benefits, even though there is a large body of research devoted to studying the relationship between gardening and health.

So, what health benefits are we most likely to obtain from gardening? A neat paper published in 2017 by Masashi Soga and colleagues from the University of Tokyo asked this question by taking seventy-six of these studies which had a similar research design and standardising their data so that they could compare the results (a so-called meta-analysis), and rank the types and amount of different health benefits obtained.[4] Even though participants were from US, Europe, Asia and the Middle East and had a wide range of socio-economic backgrounds and ages, clear findings emerged, demonstrating that regular gardeners gained broadly the same suite of positive health outcomes: reduced incidences of depression, anxiety and stress, fewer mood disturbances, improved cognitive functions, lowering of high blood pressure and reduction in Body Mass Index.

Also of interest was the finding that these benefits are not just apparent in 'healthy' people. In many cases, positive health benefits associated with gardening are even more pronounced in patients with pre-existing health conditions, particularly when they take part in horticultural therapy.[5] This is where people are prescribed gardening activities, usually (but not always) supervised by a qualified therapist as a systematic treatment. Benefits of this kind have been identified in the findings of numerous studies from the UK, US, Brazil, South Korea, Taiwan, Japan, China and the Netherlands.[6] All have found that prescribing gardening as a therapy can be an effective treatment for many conditions, including behavioural symptoms associated with diseases such as dementia[7] and schizophrenia.[8]

Gardening as a 'treatment' made me particularly curious. Even though 'green prescribing' is increasingly recognised by public health services in many countries, the term is often used vaguely. The exception to this is the practice of forest bathing – especially in Japan where this nature-based therapy has been prescribed by the health service as a medical intervention for almost forty years.[9] Japan now has over sixty accredited woodland nature-therapy trails across the country.

The success and widespread acceptance of forest bathing in Japan is largely thanks to decades of research, which gives medical practitioners the information they need in order to make a scientific judgement on prescribing it.[10] Like any drug, this includes analysis of what type of nature to prescribe, the dose, how often and for how long. Another key piece of information in making a judgement when prescribing, is knowing how successful it is compared to other drugs or interventions. This is known as its efficacy and is important because, as with all drugs, some of us will not respond to a particular treatment and alternatives will be required. And, like it or not, there are the cost implications of prescribing nature versus conventional drugs. Naturally, those holding the prescribing purse strings are particularly keen to understand this aspect. Which drugs or interventions get the same outcome but more cheaply? Even with forest bathing, knowledge of its efficacy and cost compared to other more conventional treatments is still only now emerging.

So I was keen to understand if data similar to that available for forest bathing, on prescribed dosage, efficacy and cost, exists for gardening, given how much we now know about the importance of gardening for our health.[11] My searching revealed that the process of collecting this data has only recently started, and mainly in the context of horticultural therapy. But it is revealing some important findings.

Horticultural therapy is a well-recognised health intervention which prescribes gardening for a variety of physical and mental health symptoms.[12] Sometimes the therapy sessions are guided by trained therapists; in other instances the patient is asked to follow a pre-determined walking route around a garden with volunteer guides, or self-led.[13] Indoor horticultural therapies include activities such as potting plants, or passive involvement such as viewing a garden through an open window and listening to birdsong.

Types of therapeutic gardens also vary. A number of public botanic gardens, such as the Royal Botanic Gardens in Kew, London and the New York Botanic Gardens have now broadened their purpose to include versions of therapeutic gardening activities and developed dedicated courses for teaching horticultural therapies. As well as these practices, many cities now have specifically designed therapeutic gardens, including in the UK, US, Singapore, Australia, India and a number of Scandinavian countries. Some are attached to medical facilities or public gardens, but not all. The University of Copenhagen, for example, has a nature therapy garden called Nacadia which covers approximately 1.4 hectares (3.5 acres) and contains both wildflower gardens and areas with trees.[14]

So, how effective is horticultural therapy as a treatment compared to conventional drugs and interventions? And is it more cost-effective? Both are important questions and ones that need answers before clinicians and medical administrators can start to routinely prescribe horticultural activities as an alternative to other treatments.

Ulrika Stigsdotter, a Professor of Landscape Architecture with special responsibilities in health, was one of the first to address these questions on efficiency and cost.[15] Her findings are important. She asked: how well does horticultural therapy work as a treatment for patients who are clinically stressed (to the point of being unable to work owing to their condition), compared to the more conventional treatment for this condition, cognitive behavioural therapy (CBT)? Stigsdotter's study took place over a ten-week period, and eighty-four patients were randomly assigned to either three sessions a week of a nature-based therapy session or a cognitive behavioural therapy session. The nature-based therapy involved them participating in horticultural activities in the University of Copenhagen's nature therapy garden Nacadia, with gardeners in attendance. In contrast, the cognitive behavioural therapy involved the patients undertaking two one-hour sessions each week in a clinical setting with trained psychologists, following a well-recognised cognitive behaviour stress therapy called STreSS (which stands for Specialised Treatment for Severe Bodily Stress Syndromes).

Effectiveness of the two different interventions was measured by the participants providing self-rated scores over the ten weeks on a psychological well-being index and completing a Shirom–Melamed Burnout Questionnaire (SMBQ); this asks participants to score their physical fatigue, cognitive weariness, tension and listlessness.

What they found was that both treatments worked well, with the vast majority of the patients significantly better after the ten weeks, and able to return to work. In effect, both treatments, at least after ten weeks, were effective. But one – gardening – was considerably cheaper.

But it could be argued that any outcome is only really cost-effective if the positive health outcomes are long-term. So, does one of these interventions result in better long-term outcomes? I assumed that CBT would be better because it would provide the participants with clear training on how to manage their problems by changing the way they thought and behaved. But my assumption was proved incorrect, at least in this study.

In a follow-up review of these patients covering the twelve months after their treatment, it was found that while both interventions had led to a significant decrease in the number of contacts with a medical physician, 77 per cent of those on nature-based therapy remained in work, compared to 60 per cent of those who underwent the cognitive-based therapy.[16] While this represents a small sample size and a single study, I find this really interesting because it hints that the cheaper nature-based therapy could actually be more effective in treating stress-based illnesses in the longer term – a point that is particularly pertinent when considering that in Denmark alone, treating stress-related illnesses is estimated to cost approximately 14 billion Danish kroner (£1.6 billion) a year.[17]

But are there other cost-focused studies to test whether nature-based therapies represent good economic value? Despite this being such an important question, it would appear that it has only been addressed by a few researchers to date. Those that have tackled it, however, are coming up with pretty similar findings: using nature-based interventions can result in significant cost savings compared to conventional drugs and treatments.[18]

For example, Professor Jules Pretty and Dr Jo Barton, respectively Director of the Centre of Public and Policy Engagement and leader of the Green Exercise research team at the University of Essex, calculated the costs against the benefits of 642 UK participants taking part in at least fifty hours of one of four nature-based therapies: woodland therapy, therapeutic horticulture, ecotherapy/green care and tai chi.[19] All of these activities, they found, led to large improvements in the life satisfaction and happiness scores of the participants. Using these scores, Pretty and Barton then calculated two things: first, the saving in costs from prevented visits to the doctor, a causal link routinely associated with such high happiness scores; second, increases in income from reduced sick leave, which is another well-established outcome of high happiness scores. Once the costs of delivering the nature-based courses had been added into the equation, they found that the net economic benefits of prescribing nature could be up to £31,500 per person per year.[20] This is clearly significant, both for the individuals themselves and for health service budgets.

Although there are many assumptions being made in these sorts of cost/benefit analyses, they are the same types of calculations and with the same level of detail and assumptions that are often used to make policy decisions. I therefore find this study, and others like it which also show clear cost benefits from horticultural therapy, reassuring and oddly uplifting. What they show is that interacting with nature is not only as effective for certain conditions as conventional drugs and interventions, but also highly cost effective. This is something that will please every healthcare provider.

Moving on from using horticultural therapy as a treatment, what about us as individuals pottering around our own gardens at home? For want of a better term I will call this domestic gardening – nothing to do with going out to visit a public park or nature-therapy garden, but rather the activity of gardening in our own domestic sphere. Are there some types of gardening, or particular types of gardens, that are better for us than others?

I ask this because there are many motivations for getting out into the garden, and many different types of activities gathered under the broad heading of domestic gardening. For example, we grow some plants for their beauty (ornamental horticulture), and others to eat (edible horticulture) – although some provide both, like the apple tree blossoming in spring and laden with fruit in autumn.

There are also different sorts of gardens. These include back and front gardens and even window boxes, allotment gardens (plots of land for growing produce, usually further away from our houses) and city community gardens, where communities take over ownership of small, usually neglected brownfield sites and convert them to gardens often growing a mixture of food crops and flowers. These have become a particularly welcome feature in many cities of the world in recent years. This 'taking over' can be achieved by agreement with the local authority or other body with a legal right to the land, known as community gardening, or, alternatively, by ignoring the authorities and legal rights and just doing it anyway, called guerrilla gardening.

Richard Reynolds has been a key figure in the guerrilla gardening movement. His book remains the key text, an inspiring manual of how to do something you're not really supposed to do.[21] On his website, Reynolds says he became 'an accidental activist', adding 'my pursuit has always been to normalise gardening in public space, to make the need to go guerrilla unnecessary, by proving positive impact, ideally long term'. He has certainly succeeded. His first moves to create a community of guerrilla gardeners go way back to the days of 'a world before social media' in the first years of this century. Among many other projects, he placed a riot of flowers and trees in pots and bins along Cairns Street in Toxteth, Liverpool, where many of the terraced homes were boarded up and awaiting demolition. More than a decade after he first walked the derelict pavement brandishing his trowel, his gardens are still there.

Richard's enthusiasm about his work is infectious. He is clearly committed to the benefits his idea can and does bring, and proud of what he has achieved, as he should be. Richard sent me a series of amazingly instructive 'before and after' photographs of some of his projects in London: the entrance area to Perronet House, a grey concrete block on London Road, opposite the Bakerloo Line entrance to Elephant and Castle underground station; the fragrant 'Rosemary Island' nearby; 'Lavender Fields' on Westminster Bridge Road near Lambeth North tube; pocket parks, tree pits and the neglected edges of children's playgrounds. All have been transformed. There's even a picture of Camilla, the then Duchess of Cornwall, nervously brandishing a pair of clippers with Richard grinning in the background. The picture made it into the *Sun* newspaper. This really is gardening by anyone, for everyone. Both these kinds of community gardens are on the increase in cities all over the world.

All gardens, of course, will provide the kind of benefits discussed throughout this book when we interact with them, consciously through our senses and unknowingly through hidden benefits such as enhancing our own microbiome. But what I wanted to understand was whether some types of gardening, and some types of gardens, are better for our health, and if so, why.

The first study that made me stop and think about this was, rather unexpectedly, about front gardens. I think it would be fair to say that these are probably the most unloved part of most domestic gardens. In fact, many so-called front gardens in urban areas cease to be gardens because they are paved over to become a car parking space. This has certainly happened a lot in my own neighbourhood and is being repeated in cities across the world. And this conversion to concrete is not just for parking. Outside apartment blocks, hospitals, retirement homes, offices and schools, patches of land that were formerly vegetated are 'tidied up' by covering them with paving stones and concrete. This presents a real issue for city planners, because changing from permeable soils and vegetation to impermeable concrete means that, when it rains, there is a far greater amount of surface water around, leading to localised flooding.

Strange as it may sound, evidence is now starting to suggest that front gardens are also important for our health, and our neighbours', and should ideally stay as gardens or be converted back from car parking. At least this was the finding of a team of landscape architects from the University of Sheffield who asked the question, if you convert a paved front garden back into a natural garden, what, if any, effect does it have on the people living in the house and nearby?[22] They introduced ornamental plants in pots into thirty-eight previously bare front gardens (about ten square metres, twelve square yards each) within an economically deprived region of northern England, and measured physiological and psychological indicators of stress in residents over a period of three months.[23] They also compared the before and after results with another group that did not receive plants (the control). What they found was that the group that had plants introduced into their front gardens clearly showed decreased levels of stress and improved well-being compared to the control group. Statements from the participants included that the plants made them feel more cheerful and lifted their spirits when they saw them as they came in and out.

What I also found interesting was that this better outlook on life from having flowers in the front garden was most apparent in people struggling with poor mental health. This has important implications for urban planning. Adding plants to even small areas of frontage – or even window boxes – could be an easy and important intervention to reduce stress and improve general feelings of well-being for those struggling with their mental health.

But why front gardens and not back? I think this point is illustrated perfectly in some of the interview statements from this study. When people were asked how the plants in the front gardens made them feel, they said they 'had better moods upon leaving and returning to the house'. The thing about front gardens is that we always walk past them to get into and out of our houses, schools, offices and even hospitals. So, while we might often spend a lot of time nurturing the plants in our back gardens, we probably see the front gardens more often; certainly, other people see our front gardens more. Having read this study, I suspect most of us will now think differently about the purpose of our front gardens. I certainly will, in fact I already have: the new pots of flowers are flourishing.

However, not all of us can, or want to, garden adjacent to our own homes. This is where, for the urban dweller, allotments come in.

Allotments are usually plots of land owned by a city or other organisation and leased to a group of gardeners for their exclusive use. The origin of allotments, at least in many parts of Europe, can be traced back to medieval times when large fields owned by the local lord of the manor were divided up into thin strips for individuals and families to grow food crops for their own consumption. This was called an 'open-field system', and these strips of land can still be seen today in parts of Europe. I remember being amazed when driving through north-eastern Hungary and Romania during the 1990s to still see hillsides divided into these small vertical strips of land. I'd learnt about the 'open-field system' during a brief foray into archaeology during my undergraduate degree and had assumed it was a thing of the distant past: but here it was, still happening.

The allotment system that we recognise today emerged during the nineteenth century and was closely connected to the processes of industrialisation and people moving into cites from the countryside in developing countries. Many of those that did so lived in inadequate housing, were poor and suffered from malnutrition. Allotments were therefore introduced as a system to deal with poverty and malnutrition. City administrations, churches and employers provided small plots of land for these 'landless poor' and their families to grow their own food.

Allotment provision and protection of allotment land from other urban development became legally binding in many cities in Europe during the early 1900s, and their uptake and use surged after the First and Second World Wars, particularly by returning servicemen. Even today, allotment gardening is an incredibly popular activity across the world. In the UK alone, there are currently 330,000 allotments (compared to about 1.5 million in 1918), and it has been estimated that the total number across Europe exceeds three million.

The size of allotments can vary, but typically they are between 100 square metres (120 square yards) and 250 square metres (300 square yards). In addition to crops, many allotments now also allow some ornamental plants and flowers to be grown. In some countries, however, this is still banned since it moves away from the original purpose of the allotment for growing food for personal consumption. Another recent change is in allotment ownership. Although they were originally only leased to those on lower incomes and/or who lived in housing that did not have a back garden, now all ages, generations and social economic status can and do take part in allotment gardening.

There are lots of allotments where I live in Oxford. Many of my friends have one. I don't (yet): one of the features of allotment gardening is that it is quite intensive in terms of time commitment. But of course, our principal concern here is the benefits it brings in terms of mental and physical well-being and health. So, in an entirely un-scientific one-person survey, I asked the relative of a good friend to tell me how her allotment made her feel. Her response was revealing, and deserves quoting in full:

Allotment gardening is therapy even if you aren't going through a bad time. When I first got my allotment I felt revitalised because I had a purpose: this plot of land would only flourish if I was prepared to nurture it. There's nothing more fantastic than growing things, planting the seeds, feeling the earth in your hands and then watching the seedlings grow. It's amazing and extremely rewarding. You begin with an allotment plot which is in a state and you gradually transform it into a garden oasis. And no matter if something goes wrong and won't grow there's always next year to have another go. The lettuce or carrots might wilt and die one year but they're fine the next. You might mistakenly plant ten courgette plants the first summer and then be inundated with hundreds of courgettes later on but you soon learn! The allotment is never boring to me, I'm constantly discovering new things and challenging myself. You gain confidence as you learn to grow from cuttings and share gardening tips with neighbouring allotment holders – it's very sociable. And if I'm on my own I never feel lonely as I'm surrounded by the birds and the insects as I weed or dig. I take my toddler son down to the allotment and it's so much fun for him, he rolls about in the mud, helps to carry the vegetables and just loves being there. I hope it'll rub off and he'll love gardening when he's older. The allotment is so good for my mind and my body as it demands I work at it all year round, in all weather, freezing or hot. It keeps my Vit D levels high. When I leave the allotment, I feel rejuvenated and rested – and sometimes frustrated because there's always more to be done. But that's what I love about it.

This quote really captures it all for me. Even if we don't know the science behind what is going on in our bodies when we garden or tend our allotment, we do know that it makes us feel better – both while tending the plants, and also for hours and sometimes days afterwards. One of the things I've found so satisfying about researching this book is finding that the science backs up our instincts about interacting with nature – it not only *feels* like it is doing us good, mentally and physically, it actually *is* doing us good.

So far, I've treated the discussion of different kinds of urban garden separately. I think it would be impossible (and not particularly useful) to ask whether some sorts of activities – planting, weeding, pruning – are better than others, because they are all interlinked. However, the places we garden have been investigated by researchers to see if some are better for our health.[24]

To investigate the relevant health benefits of gardening in allotments compared to domestic gardens, a team of researchers led by Christopher Young from the Swiss Federal Research Unit for Forest, Snow and Landscape Research in Zürich, Switzerland, interviewed over 300 participants in the city. These were made up of two groups: those who gardened in a plot attached to their own home (domestic gardens), and those who gardened on an allotment.

The interview, in the form of an in-person discussion or filling in an online questionnaire, contained questions designed to assess the impact of their garden/allotment on their psychological well-being. In particular, the researchers measured the participants' levels of stress and recovery attention restoration by asking questions specifically related to two theories in environmental psychology: that being in natural environments promotes recovery from stress;

and that it also engages our involuntary attention, thereby allowing recovery of a fatigued directed attention.[25] For example, the participants were asked to state their level of agreement, from 'strongly agree' to 'strongly disagree', with statements such as 'My garden gives me a good break from my day-to-day routine' and 'In my garden my attention is drawn to many interesting things'.

The participants were also asked about garden-related stress. In this case they were asked to say how strongly they agreed or disagreed with the statement 'I often feel under pressure when I think of the tasks that need doing in my garden'. In addition to collecting responses to the questionnaires, data on possible factors that might explain the participants' responses were also collected. These included, for example, the distance of the allotments from the participants' houses, and the number of different plant species in each garden/allotment. These potential explanatory variables were then used in the modelling to try and tease out what features might be responsible for any preference for allotments or back gardens that emerged.

The findings were not what I expected. I had assumed that boring-looking allotments some distance from home and with little colour would be less beneficial to mental well-being, and that participants' reactions to domestic gardening would be far more positive. In fact, it was the other way around. Even when controlling for socio-economic factors such as age, gender, employment and job-level status, people gardening in allotments felt less stressed and their attention more restored after doing so. Why?

The second surprising finding to me was that the number of different plant species was higher in allotments than in gardens. And it would appear that this was the best explanatory variable for why people felt mentally better in these spaces. This relationship between higher levels of plant biodiversity and better mental well-being has been demonstrated before, but largely, as discussed in Chapter 3, in the context of public gardens and large colourful displays of flowers.[26] What I found surprising was that the same is true of allotments. Having thought about it a bit more, I came to realise that the mixture of edible and ornamental plants typically grown on an allotment might well account for these higher levels of biodiversity and, therefore, the benefits associated with seeing different shapes and colours.

Third and finally, I was surprised by the finding that not all gardening is rosy (if you'll pardon the pun). Around 16 per cent of gardeners, most of them domestic gardeners, reported garden-related stress associated with the amount of work needed to keep the garden tidy.

There are a number of important considerations for urban policies emerging from this study, especially if these findings are shown to be reproduced elsewhere. As acknowledged by the authors, making further provision for allotments in cities could be an important tool to reduce income- and health-related inequalities.[27] This is because those typically using allotments, at least in Zürich but probably in many other cities as well, were from less well-off groups and/or residents of apartment blocks, and yet they gain the same, if not more, mental well-being benefits from allotment gardening as they would from a domestic garden. Another consideration is what to do about domestic gardens that cause stress for the homeowners? Possibly we now need to start to think about ways to encourage greater sharing of domestic gardens, so that they become a benefit to many, rather than a burden for some.

This idea of sharing gardens and gardening activities is nothing new, of course. Over the past forty years or so, and increasingly in the past few years, community gardens have sprung up in many cities across the world. These are different from allotments because the gardening duties and horticultural produce are shared. People come together as a community, garden together and share the vegetables, fruits and flowers that it yields. Community gardens are also now found in many schools either as a 'club', where pupils and staff garden together, or as part of a weekly activity in the school curriculum. Land is usually owned by a public body and access provided communally, for example in the shared outdoor space of a block of flats, or outside a community centre or school.

So, does community gardening provide the same sort of positive benefits as allotments or private, domestic gardens? The few studies to have compared community gardening to other gardening activities to date suggest that they may do even better.[28,29] First, they provide greater social interactions, reducing loneliness, isolation and improving mental well-being.[30] Second, people actively engaged in community gardening appear to have higher levels of optimism and mental resilience from stress than those who do other non-gardening and outdoor social activities. And third, working in a community garden can improve the nutritional behaviours of those participating, with an increase in the consumption of fruit and vegetables.[31] This finding has particularly significant implications given the importance of a good microbiome in our gut for both short- and long-term health benefits, something strongly influenced by both diet (more fruit and vegetables grown organically) and being immersed in nature (Chapter 7). Growing our own provides us with both.

If you've stayed with me on this journey this far, you might be forgiven for feeling a bit confused about what are the best activities to do outdoors, especially taking this chapter and the previous one together. There seem to be many instances where a small change in our outdoor activities can make quite a big difference to our health. But it leaves lots of questions about exactly how: where to walk, whether to walk, sit or run, for how long, what to see, touch, hear, smell? Where to garden, front or back, allotment or community garden? Even writing this list makes me feel a bit stressed.

Pulling these different strands of evidence together is difficult, so I was particularly relieved to find a synthesis of many of these published studies carried out in 2021 by a team of researchers led by Dr Peter Coventry from the department of Health Sciences at the University of York.[32] In this, they were effectively addressing the question that I wanted answered: are some outdoor activities interacting with nature better for our health than others?

Coventry and his team screened 14,321 published academic papers about health outcomes associated with individual or group-based activities undertaken in outdoor green (and blue) spaces. From these, they selected fifty studies that had a similar research design, meaning that their results could be compared and contrasted in a meta-analysis. Activities that were considered alongside each other included: social and therapeutic gardening activities; care farming that involves the use of agricultural landscape and farming practices; environmental conservation activities; exercise in green space; nature-based therapies for stress relief such as forest bathing and mindfulness; and nature-based arts and craft tasks that involve being in nature and using natural materials to construct artefacts.

Reassuringly, their meta-analysis found that across all activities, outdoor nature-based interventions improved mental health. And this occurred in all groups studied, including older adults with long-term conditions, those with common mental health problems and serious mental illnesses such as schizophrenia and bipolar disorder, as well as in healthy adults.

The implications of this finding are hugely important for healthcare policies. It shows that any nature-based outdoor activity will have a positive impact on our mental health; also, that nature-based interventions are effective both in managing pre-existing mental health problems, and as a preventative measure to keep people well.[33] The largest positive effects were found in forest therapies and group gardening therapies, especially those that last for twelve weeks or more. Green exercise was also associated with reducing depressive symptoms. Even though exercise indoors can also do this, it is known that additional benefits can be gained from exercising in nature, as evidenced here.[34]

Regardless of the type of activity, they also found that to be most effective, the interventions need to last at least eight to twelve weeks (more if possible) and take 90–120 minutes a week, divided into sessions of a minimum of twenty minutes per session.

These same numbers keep coming up in many studies, as we saw in the previous chapter – and I have found them remarkably helpful in turning academic abstractions into daily routine. Twenty minutes is longer than I used to take walking the dogs or cycling to work. I have now extended these daily activities with another spin round the park (to my dogs' initial confusion) or a different, longer (and nicer) commute. I have also changed my route, so the last part includes walking through the park. Do I feel better for it? Possibly – but then it is hard to tell with a sample size of one and given that I already know the potential outcome of the experiment. What I therefore find particularly reassuring about these types of meta-analyses, many of which have been cited in this book, is that they are assessing the data from literally hundreds of studies involving thousands of participants.[35] And yet all are showing the same thing. Being outdoors in nature, for at least twenty minutes, three or four times a week, provides a whole host of health benefits to young and old alike, healthy and unhealthy, and in both the short and long term.

No more excuses. Gardening is something that we should definitely timetable into our busy lives.

Prescribing Nature: For Self, Health and Wealth

I had no idea when I started researching this book how personal it would all become. I have never written a book or paper before which has changed my own activities this way. I now have four diffusers in my house, puffing out various scents: lavender in my bedroom, rosemary in my study and hinoki and cedar oils in two other rooms. The number of houseplants has trebled, and yellow and green cut flowers in vases adorn many surfaces. Hellebore plants with their green petals are now proudly blooming in the garden, alongside a diversity of different colours, shapes and structures. I care less about how neat the garden looks and more about how many different shapes, shades of green and colours I can see. With this diversity of planting, songbirds are now abundant – and I take time to listen to them every morning. I now also see the lawn as an 'add-on', not the focus of the garden – and if it is a bit patchy here and there, I simply refuse to let this stress me (or my husband). I hope that the environmental microbiome has also increased from my efforts to increase diversity and not use chemical fertilisers. I no longer wear gardening gloves – soil under my nails is fine. And my front garden is now full of pots with colourful flowers.

So, what about the city around me, which is less under my control?

I am constantly reading and hearing the statement 'we need more green spaces' in articles and speeches by academics, policy makers, healthcare practitioners and non-government organisations. But what exactly is meant by this?

Green space is a term which has come to mean many different things to many different people. It has even become a target in the United Nations Biological Diversity Framework, signed by 189 countries in Montreal in 2022, which makes the commitment that every signatory will 'Significantly increase the area and quality and connectivity of, access to, and benefits from green [and blue] spaces in urban and densely populated areas... improving human health and well-being and connection to nature...' I see a danger here. While I strongly support the drive for more green spaces, I think it is important to recognise that not all green spaces are equal. They need to be of the right quality, in the right place, and not simply moved when considered in the wrong place.

Take for example an idea called 'biodiversity offsetting' which is catching on in countries across the world. This is a policy that allows developers to build offices and homes on green spaces provided they agree to create an equivalent area of green space, of a higher biodiversity value, elsewhere in the city or, more often than not, somewhere outside of the city. This policy might be good for certain types of rare and endangered wildlife, with money and effort flowing into new habitat creation, but it totally loses sight of the fact that green spaces in cities, of the right type and in the right place, provide critical services for human health and well-being. The right place means within a maximum of fifteen minutes' walking distance of one's home. If people have to walk further than this or have to catch a bus or drive to access green space, they simply won't do so.

If the green space in cities is low-grade and is not providing the right sorts of nature for our health, then we should enhance it, plant additional new species and create the necessary ecological processes for wildlife to thrive; not cover it in concrete and hope nature will provide the same services elsewhere. It won't. We need to think of nature as an infrastructure underpinning human well-being in cities and urban areas, across the world.

And yet, in writing this book, the point that has really come home to me is that we also don't need to wait for urban planners and politicians to create the ideal green spaces and prescribe that we spend time in them. We now know enough to self-prescribe in our homes, offices or working spaces, gardens, allotments and when out walking. However small these individual actions might be, they have the potential to provide a large number of health benefits overall. And we need to be encouraging others to do the same.

This is already catching on in schools in the UK. Many make gardening a weekly classroom activity, and a number of organisations are arguing for it to form part of the curriculum, not least because it teaches children about where food comes from. But I personally feel that we need be careful on this one. Once it becomes a formal 'school activity' for some children, and especially teenagers, this could have the opposite effect – and instead not provide the health benefits we want to see or instil longer term habits of interacting with nature.

I say this after reflecting on the studies mentioned at the beginning of Chapter 10. When asked, people didn't say they garden for its health benefits, but rather because they enjoy it. Gardening for children needs to remain a fun activity that is relaxing and enjoyable – not something that they are going to be tested and graded on at the end of the year. And for teenagers in particular, working and enjoying time in nature needs to be seen as something 'cool'. This is why I really like and support the 'guerrilla gardening' movements in London and other cities across the world.[1] They are inspiring teenagers and young people to interact with plants and turning ugly public concrete spaces into patches of nature, teeming with wildlife. This is occurring in some of the most economically deprived areas of these cities – but without a single textbook or concept of teacher-led activity in sight.

While on the subject of young people, another thing I kept noticing when looking at studies for this book was how effective interacting with nature appears to be for children's health and cognitive performance. There are now thousands of studies with strong scientific evidence demonstrating these effects in children. In 2021 a really nice meta-analysis attempted to synthesise their findings by examining data from around 300 of these, finding that exposure to green space produced an overall 147 per cent improvement in health and cognitive outcomes in children.[2] With this sort of quantitative evidence, outdoor classrooms and forest schools take on a whole new significance; even though many have been arguing the case for years, they are still often seen as a niche form of education. We really must now take note of this sort of evidence and actively green the walls, playgrounds and classrooms of every school. By not doing so we are doing a disservice to our children and storing up a whole host of unnecessary health and educational problems.

But what about the more formal side of prescribing nature by medics – as a 'drug' for those who already have a set of identified health issues? Are we now at the point where we can prescribe nature as a replacement to conventional drugs and interventions? Sadly, I think, not yet. As mentioned in Chapter 10, to prescribe nature there needs to be evidence on the efficacy and dose of nature, and proper clinical trials to enable direct comparison with conventional drugs and interventions. Here there is still a large scientific knowledge gap. Admittedly, some information is already available, for example to enable the prescription of forest bathing. This is also the case for some types of horticultural therapy. But with this latter practice, it is still heavily reliant on volunteers and garden staff to deliver the necessary spaces and activities, often without a healthcare practitioner in sight. It also still doesn't have the widespread recognition across the medical profession that it probably deserves to have.

For most clinicians, nature is still seen as an extra, an additional 'add-on': important certainly, but far from realising its full potential for improving health. Nor have we engaged sufficiently robustly with the potential of nature for preventing us getting sick in the first place.

Using nature to help reduce the incidence and severity of common and serious conditions could have huge benefits for health service providers across the world, as they struggle with ever more complex demands and ever-increasing competition for resources.

Having said this, a large number of organisations, including national health services, NGOs and charities, are now providing guidance, handbooks and marked trails and spaces designed specifically to enable healthcare practitioners to 'prescribe' routes and activities where patients can interact with nature. Activities under this heading include exercising or walking in nearby parks or attending other formal outdoor activity programmes.[3] There are also now a number of medical practitioner handbooks and dedicated nature prescription websites available in the UK, US, Canada, and elsewhere.[4]

While many of these are excellent, they are still very general in their advice and focus. They are often missing recommendations on what specific aspects of nature to interact with, particularly in relation to certain plant smells and sensing a diverse environmental microbiome. Perhaps the science on these topics is still too new – but I fear there is also a tendency to only think about visual aspects of nature, with sound as a poor relation and smell mentioned as an afterthought, if at all. If the emerging evidence I have come across and discussed in this book is correct, the list of what and how we sense nature for our health should possibly be the other way around: smell, sound, sight, in this order.

There are also remarkably few websites or practical guides on the use of biophilic design for indoor settings and the type of nature that we should have in our houses, schools and office spaces to gain its health benefits and reduce the effects of sick building syndrome. There is therefore an urgent need for far more links to be made between the scientific evidence base demonstrating the specific types of nature that are best for specific ailments, both outdoors and indoors, and the type and dose of nature that should be prescribed.

So how do we do this? How do we fit all the current scientific evidence of what happens when we see, hear, smell and touch nature and its environmental microbiome into some sort of 'prescribing' pathway, so that a specific set of nature interactions can be recommended for a particular condition? I have pondered this question many times while writing this book. Then I came across a paper reporting the outputs from a workshop in 2016 in which a group of scientists asked this same question about the functions of green space.[5] What they came up with were three general headings for how green space can be used to improve human health: *reducing harm* (e.g. reducing exposure to air pollution, noise and heat); *restoring capacities* (e.g. attention restoration and physiological stress recovery); and *building capacities* (e.g. encouraging physical activity and facilitating social cohesion).

I find these headings incredibly useful. They add clarity and can be adapted to create prescribing pathways for aligning which aspects of sensory interaction with nature can be used for what types of conditions.

Under the first heading, for example, hearing birdsong has been shown to reduce post-operative pain. We also experience less eye-fatigue when we look at wooden panelling compared to plaster walls or concrete. These interactions reduce harm. So too does the reduction in our blood pressure, adrenaline hormones and heart-rate variability that we get when see certain colours and shapes of nature, quantifiably demonstrating physiological and psychological calming. These interactions reduce the harm that is associated with high levels of stress and anxiety.

Under heading two, restoration capacities identified for green space are pretty much the same as those for many other aspects of nature (e.g. attention restoration and physiological stress recovery) – but the difference here is that these capacities can also be restored by seeing, hearing and smelling certain types of nature not just in outdoor green space, but also by encountering nature indoors. We have seen that viewing plants on our desk can provide a restorative mental mini-break, and that the scent of, for example, coniferous timber linings in rooms can do this too. Smelling rosemary and mint is also shown to keep us more awake and alert when undertaking difficult tasks.

However, it is heading three, building capacities, where I believe the greatest untapped potential health benefits associated with interacting with nature lie. The authors of the meta-study list the building capacities of green space as 'encouraging physical activity and facilitating social cohesion'. This is correct and appropriate. But nature can offer us much more, and we need to add to this list. Two sensory interactions in particular deserve more detailed study in this respect: smell and interacting with the environmental microbiome.

As noted in Chapter 4, smelling certain scents from the Cupressaceae family can significantly raise levels of natural killer cells, which attack cancers and viruses in our blood. This contributes to building long-term health capacities in ways that we have yet to fully realise and capture in how we use nature. So too does the potential of smelling limonene to reduce inflammation in the respiratory tract. As also discussed in Chapter 4, it has been shown to enhance anti-allergenic and anti-inflammatory compounds in our blood and inhibit inflammatory cells and other inflammation pathways in the lungs, reducing airway hyper-responsiveness, a characteristic feature of asthma, bronchitis and chronic obstructive pulmonary disease. These are clear examples of the potential for building long-term health capacities through a specific, practical interaction with nature. We need to bring this insight much more clearly into focus.

Similarly, interacting with a diverse environmental microbiome can not only significantly improve our own skin and gut microbiome, but also trigger the production of secondary metabolites and other compounds in our blood with the potential to positively influence a plethora of autoimmune and anti-inflammatory responses.

Both of these interactions, smelling certain plant scents and interacting with diverse environmental microbiomes, therefore have huge and as yet largely untapped potential to enhance our own immune systems and build capacity and resilience to some of the biggest causes of death from non-communicable diseases, all across the world.

The science associated with the health benefits that we gain from sensing many aspects of nature is young but growing quickly. We need to act now to start to use this type of framing to kick-start the types of clinical testing and human trials necessary for such interactions with nature to become a viable prescribed alternative to conventional drugs and interventions for a range of conditions. We also need to build it into public health spatial planning processes, so that identification of important areas for nature in cities for health are pre-determined and not, as happens too often, added as an afterthought, if at all.[6]

Twenty years from now, I hope it will be unnecessary to say this. Instead, interacting with nature in specific ways beneficial for our health will be a routine part of the prescribing process formal and informal, for a range of physical and mental conditions and social challenges. It may even have resulted in improved population-level health outcomes – and it will be cheaper than business as usual.

This leads me on to my very last point – prescribing nature for wealth. Using nature to reduce harm, restore capacities and build capacities in our health has the potential to save billions of pounds from global health budgets, even if only a tiny fraction of the estimates made thus far on this topic are correct. Health economists are already starting to ask the right questions about nature – but again, they need the sorts of efficacy/cost trials comparing nature interactions to conventional drug effectiveness/costs described in Chapter 10. These sorts of trials are still very scarce, but are essential if cost is the driver.

Yet there is something that makes me uncomfortable putting this sort of price on nature, and I am not alone in this. Why? Because nature is far more than just something that is useful for our health. It is not a dispensable commodity. It is an inherent part of us and provides multiple known and unknown ecosystem services.[7] We cannot survive without a diverse nature around us. I strongly believe that access to nature and the multiple benefits it provides is a human right – in the same way that we demand rights to fresh air, clean water, access to education, transport and health facilities. Everyone should have a right to access biodiverse nature. Rich, poor, young, old, ill, healthy.

Now is the time to stop thinking of nature as 'nice to have' and at the bottom of the priority list in urban infrastructure development. We must see it as an essential aspect of providing health and well-being and other multiple benefits to those people who will live, work and go to school in these new developments. Remember that by 2050, 70 per cent of us will be living in urban environments. Nature provides us with untold wealth. It is priceless and we must protect and enhance it – we need nature more than it needs us.

Acknowledgements

Writing acknowledgements for any book is always a bit of a minefield – if you are not careful it can just end up being one long list sounding like an end-of-term speech day – and yet inadvertently missing out thanking someone you really should have done. But these acknowledgements are particularly difficult. I say this because to be able to write a book like this, spanning so many scientific disciplines, and covering many topics that are long way outside my own area of expertise, relied on me calling in many favours from colleagues, friends and sometimes people I had only heard of, and, to this day, never met.

'Would you mind just fact-checking this bit for me?' became a constant opening sentence to many emails, and I need to thank all the long-suffering and tolerant scientists who received these emails from me. There are too many to name them all, but I would like to especially thank St Edmund Hall colleague and friend Dr Robert Wilkins, who is Director of the Biomedical Sciences Course in the Medical Sciences Division at Oxford University. He used his own knowledge and that of colleagues in his medical sciences networks to fact-check a number of the medical sections. I'd also like to thank Professor Paul Harvey, former Head of the Biology Department at Oxford and eminent ecologist. He has one of the most brilliant minds and is someone not afraid to give honest, tough criticism. Paul 'kicked the tyres' on all chapters in the first draft of this book and I remain indebted to him for his time, patience and scientific scrutiny and assurance in the early stages of writing this book.

I'd also like to thank members of my lab group in Oxford and in particular Eva Herreros-Moya, who read a first draft, again providing really helpful and insightful comments. Professor Tim Coulson, a fellow author and current Head of the Department of Biology at Oxford, picked up the baton of scientific reading for the last draft; then a literary legend for many academic scientists, Dr Andrew Sugden, took on the final shift in reading the proof. Andrew, who is a long-time friend and colleague, was Deputy Editor and International Managing Editor for many years at *Science* magazine. Andrew's editorial red pencil is something that any scientist who has published in *Science* will know only too well. I am therefore deeply grateful to him for coming out of retirement to wield the red pencil once again.

Writing in a non-academic style is something that I think is difficult for the majority of scientists. If that is not bad enough, having to bring in-person experiences and reflections can sometimes feel like one step too far! I am therefore deeply grateful to a second set of people who dragged me, sometimes kicking and screaming, or at least with much resistance, over the threshold of 'writing for scientists' to 'writing for everyone'. Rebecca Carter, my wonderful agent, started me on this journey, to be followed by my cousin Marion Dodson-Paul, who is herself an excellent policy writer, and then my long-time close friend and former newspaper journalist, Joanna Gibbon. All helped me hugely in this respect. Joanna even stepped in to do some of interviews published in the book – realising that I would get there in the end, but it would probably be quicker and less painful for us both if she did it for me. Once the first full draft was written, the skills, patience and writing-style genius of my editor Alexis Kirshbaum, and Non-Fiction Publishing Director, Ian Marshall, both at Bloomsbury, came to the forefront. I feel privileged to have worked with them and their wonderful team and am indebted to them.

Given the topic of this book I was extremely keen to have photos and at least some figures – but again, those that I would normally put in a scientific textbook, needed some radical rethinking. Working with Lauren Whybrow, Managing Editorial Director at Bloomsbury, has therefore been a total delight. Her guidance over this aspect of the book has been exemplary and again, I have personally learnt so much from working with her. Knowing who to ask to do the figures, however, was easy because one of the many things I learnt when working at Kew, was that they have a superb designer, Jeff Eden. Jeff can turn the most boring scientific graph into something that anyone can immediately understand, and he has once again worked his magic on the figures in this book – and if they still look at bit 'too scientific' this is entirely my fault. I am deeply grateful to him.

There are two other people who I cannot easily fit into the categories above, but need to thank and these are Dr

Richard Deverell and Baroness Rosie Boycott. Although both have also provided support on style and content (Richard read two drafts of the book), they have provided something additional – and that is belief in me and my ability to deliver it. Richard and I worked closely together when I was at Kew – he was my boss – and he has remained someone who is incredibly supportive and provides a level of assurance that I find extremely helpful. Although I have only come to know Rosie in the past two years in the House of Lords, she is someone that I have come to see as an exceptional colleague and friend.

Finally, to the very personal part. None of this from the first page onwards would have been possible without the love and support of my family – my husband Andrew, and my children Alice, James and Harry. They have literally 'lived' this book, and some of the first inklings to write this and explore the topics described herein, came about from my interactions on many holidays and weekends spent stomping in the fields and countryside both in the UK and beyond. When the children were small, Andrew always insisted every Saturday we went out walking in green spaces – even if pouring with rain and everyone was grumpy – because he observed that within twenty minutes of being outdoors everyone would be in much happier place mood-wise. And he was right. Our family thrived being outdoors in a way that simply didn't happen if we went to the cinema or some other indoor event. This observation led to us buying a tent and spending a number of holidays driving around Europe, spending time in some of the most beautiful landscapes – an outdoor habit we then took to explore the wonderful national parks in the US and Canada. At the time, I viewed these holidays as being restorative and happy because we were all away together – but, funnily enough, spending time in a villa with a pool (which we did once) was not the same success. Researching for this book has made me realise why, but it took me spending time outdoors in green spaces with my wonderful family to first understand this, and this book is dedicated to them.

Further explanation of the graphs

A more detailed explanation of the science shown in each of the graphs, along with the source of the research.

Page 23: Twelve-month progress in superior working memory for school children who encounter the lowest third (low) and highest third (high) levels of greenness within the school boundaries. 'Visit' refers to number of the three-monthly tests which occurred over the school year 2012– 2013. Shading represents the 95 per cent confidence limits (error bars or estimated range of values) in the data. Dadvand, P. et al., 'Green spaces and cognitive development in primary schoolchildren', *Proceedings of the National Academy of Sciences* **112**, pp. 7937–42 (2015).

Page 28: Different tree forms and resulting canopy shapes.

Page 34: Fractal dimensions of the horizons of different landscapes: (a) coniferous forest in Canada; (b) savanna landscape in Kenya; (c) Chicago's skyline.

Page 90: (a) Measuring different monoterpenes in the atmosphere of Tsubetsu coniferous forest (*Picea jezoensis, Abies sachalinensis*) in Japan using gas chromatography. Each peak indicates the relative intensity of different volatile organic compounds in the ambient air. Note the arrow illustrating the high concentrations of α-pinene (peak 2) in the coniferous forest; (b) the relative amount of this compound in the participant's blood before walking; and the large increase (c) after walking for sixty minutes in the forest. Sumitomo, K. et al., 'Conifer-derived monoterpenes and forest walking', *Mass Spectrometry* **4**, A0042-A0042 (2015).

Page 97: This experiment was to understand the effects of smelling increased concentrations of α-pinene and limonene on two measures of physiological calming, alpha brainwave activity and heart-rate variability, and showed a strong relationship in both measures. As concentrations of α-pinene and limonene increase, calming effect increases in all participants, both male and female. Ikei, H., C. Song, and Y. Miyazaki, *Effects of olfactory stimulation by α-pinene on autonomic nervous activity.* Journal of Wood Science, 2016. **62**(6): p. 568-572.

Page 101: Before and after measurements of adrenaline hormone (in participants' urine) and natural killer cells (in their blood) following three nights of sleeping in rooms where air was infused with volatile organic compounds from the Hinoki cypress tree. The results were statistically strong, demonstrating that after three nights there was: (a) a decrease in the stress hormone adrenaline; (b) increased levels of activity and percentage of natural killer cells. Li, Q. et al., 'Effect of phytoncide from trees on human natural killer cell function', *International Journal of Immunopathology and Pharmacology* 22, pp. 951–9 (2009).

Page 122: Mean effect sizes of natural sounds on health and positive affective outcomes, and stress and annoyance outcomes for different types of natural sounds. A positive mean value (to the right of the dashed zero line) indicates health and positive affective outcomes improved in groups exposed to natural sound, and a negative value (to the left of the dashed zero line) indicates stress and annoyance indicators decreased in groups exposed to natural sound. Buxton, R. T., Pearson, A. L., Allou, C., Fristrup, K. & Wittemyer, G., 'A synthesis of health benefits of natural sounds and their distribution in national parks', *Proceedings of the National Academy of Sciences* **118**, e2013097118 (2021).

Page 125: Acoustic signature of birdsong of the (a) European robin (Erithacus rubecula) and (b) carrion crow (Corvus corone) – note the differences in harmonic pattern and complexity in the two songs.

Page 130: Mean pain score of sixty patients recovering from an operation during ninety minutes after the event. The control group heard no sounds but wore headphones, the intervention group wore headphones and heard sounds of nature. Saadatmand, V. et al., 'Effects of natural sounds on pain: A randomized controlled trial with patients receiving mechanical ventilation support', *Pain Management Nursing* **16**, pp. 483–92 (2015).

Page 171: These show the apparent association between two global megatrends in biodiversity and public health. (a) Declining biodiversity since 1970 as measured by three indices. LI, Living Plant Index; WBI, World Bird Index; WPSI, Waterbird Population Status Index (Butchart et al, 2010); (b) Increasing trends in the prevalence of inflammatory diseases. Asthma and allergic rhinitis among military conscripts from 1966 to 2003 (Latvala et al, 2005) are shown as an example. Von Hertzen, L., Hanski, I. & Haahtela, T., 'Natural immunity: biodiversity loss and inflammatory diseases are two global megatrends that might be related', *EMBO Reports* 12, pp. 1089–93 (2011).

Page 180: Comparison of skin microbiota and bloods of children who played in the two types of sand pits over the period of the twenty-eight days of the experiment; (a) showing significant increase in the richness of the four major groups of 'good' microbiota on the skin of the children who played in the seeded sandpit (intervention) compared to sterile sandpit (placebo) group; (b) mean change (increase) in good t-cells (A) in the bloods of intervention group and (decrease) in bad t-cells B) compared to the placebo group. Roslund, Marja I., et al., 'A Placebo-controlled double-blinded test of the biodiversity hypothesis of immune-mediated diseases: Environmental microbial diversity elicits changes in cytokines and increase in T regulatory cells in young children', *Ecotoxicology and Environmental Safety*.

Page 199: The comparison of the skin biota of office participants who sat in a room containing a green wall for twenty days, compared to those in a control room with no green wall, showed significant differences. Those who were in the room with the green wall developed a much higher abundance of 'good' types of bacteria, known to be positive for skin health (*Lactobacillus*) on their skin. They also showed significant lowering of markers in the blood that are associated with causing inflammation and associated inflammatory diseases. Soininen, L., et al. 'Indoor green wall affects health-associated commensal skin microbiota and enhances immune regulation: a randomized trial among urban office workers', Scientific Reports 12, 1-9 (2022).

Illustration Credits

'Queen of the Night' tulip: Courtesy of Liv Meinert / Pixabay; Common buttercup: © Nigel Cattlin / Alamy Stock Photo; Blue hydrangeas (acidic soils): © Moment/ Getty Images; Blue hydrangeas (alkaline soils): © RM Floral / Alamy Stock Photo

'Flowers in a Terracotta Vase' by Jan van Huysum © The National Gallery, London. All rights reserved

Black walnut: © imageBROKER.com GmbH & Co. KG / Alamy Stock Photo; Red oak: © iStock / Getty Images Plus; Easter white pine: © Zoonar GmbH / Alamy Stock Photo; Southern yellow pine: © iStock / Getty Images Plus; Cross-hatches of trees: These illustrations come from *Understanding Wood* by R. Bruce Hoadley, used courtesy of Taunton Press and Active Media Group

The Garden of Eden: © Christie's Images / Bridgeman Images

Sir Hugh Plat: © The History Collection / Alamy Stock Photo; Anthrium © Florilegius / Bridgeman Images; Peace lily © Florilegius / Bridgeman Images

Swedish living room: Courtesy Värmlands Museum

Green wall at St Edmund Hall, University of Oxford: © John Cairns, photograph by John Cairns; Seoul's City Hall: © Andia / Alamy Stock Photo; Office experiment: From Yin, J. et al., 'Effects of biophilic indoor environment on stress and anxiety recovery: A between-subjects experiment in virtual reality', Environment International 136, 105427 (2020), used under Creative Commons licence CC BY 4.0.

Victoria Park, Leicester: © charistoone-images / Alamy Stock Photo; Victoria Park, Portsmouth: © Nigel Cattlin / Alamy Stock Photo, © Nigel Cattlin / Alamy Stock Photo; Original plans for New York's Central Park: ©Odonovanshn/ Shutterstock.com

'The Mall' in Central Park, 1901: © Universal History Archive / Getty Images; 'The Mall' in Central Park, present day: © iStock / Getty Images Plus

Maidenhair tree: © Paul Wood / Alamy Stock Photo; Maidenhair tree detail: © imageBROKER.com GmbH & Co. KG / Alamy Stock Photo; Plane tree detail: © Erik Koole / Alamy Stock Photo; Plane tree: © iStock / Getty Images Plus; American sweet gum: © Buiten-Beeld / Alamy Stock Photo; American sweet gum detail: © Steffen Hauser / botanikfoto / Alamy Stock Photo

CDL's Tree House in Singapore: © Arcaid Images / Alamy Stock Photo

Green wall in Colombia: Images courtesy of Ignacio Solano and Paisajismo Urbano

All images of guerrilla gardening: © Richard Reynolds

Images on page 34: Courtesy of jplenio/ Pixabay; Courtesy of djsudermann/ Pixabay; © 4kclips/ Shutterstock.com

Notes

INTRODUCTION

1 Ulrich, R. S., 'View through a window may influence recovery from surgery', *Science* 224, pp. 420–1 (1984).

2 Wilson, E. O., *Biophilia*, Harvard University Press, Harvard, 1984.

3 Joye, Y. & Van den Berg, A., 'Is love for green in our genes? A critical analysis of evolutionary assumptions in restorative environments research', *Urban Forestry & Urban Greening* 10, pp. 261–8 (2011).

4 Miyazaki, Y., *Shinrin Yoku: The Japanese Art of Forest Bathing*, Timber Press, Portland, 2018; Li, Q., *Shinrin-Yoku: The Art and Science of Forest Bathing*, Penguin UK, London, 2018.

5 Hansen, M. M., Jones, R. & Tocchini, K., 'Shinrin-Yoku (Forest Bathing) and Nature Therapy: A State-of-the-Art Review', *International Journal of Environmental Research and Public Health* 14, doi:10.3390/ijerph14080851 (2017).

6 Sarkar, C., Webster, C. & Gallacher, J., 'Residential greenness and prevalence of major depressive disorders: a cross-sectional, observational, associational study of 94,879 adult UK Biobank participants', *The Lancet Planetary Health* 2, e162–e173 (2018).

7 Donovan, G. H. et al., 'The relationship between trees and human health: evidence from the spread of the emerald ash borer', *American Journal of Preventive Medicine* 44, pp. 139–45 (2013).

I GREEN HORIZONS

1 Owens, M., 'Capability Brown Is the Landscape Designer Behind England's Most Iconic Gardens', *Architectural Digest*, via https://www.architecturaldigest.com/story/capability-brown-landscape-design-england

2 Li, D. & Sullivan, W. C., 'Impact of views to school landscapes on recovery from stress and mental fatigue', *Landscape and Urban Planning* 148, pp. 149–58 (2016).

3 Lee, K. E., Williams, K. J., Sargent, L. D., Williams, N. S. & Johnson, K. A., '40-second green roof views sustain attention: The role of micro-breaks in attention restoration', *Journal of Environmental Psychology* 42, pp. 182–9 (2015).

4 O'Connor, D. B., Thayer, J. F. & Vedhara, K., 'Stress and health: A review of psychobiological processes', *Annual Review of Psychology* 72, pp. 663–88 (2021).

5 Song, C., Ikei, H. & Miyazaki, Y., 'Physiological effects of visual stimulation with forest imagery', *International Journal of Environmental Research and Public Health* 15, p. 213 (2018).

6 Brown, D. K., Barton, J. L. & Gladwell, V. F., 'Viewing nature scenes positively affects recovery of autonomic function following acute-mental stress', *Environmental Science & Technology* 47, pp. 5,562–9 (2013).

7 Ulrich, R. S. et al., 'Stress recovery during exposure to natural and urban environments', *Journal of Environmental Psychology* 11, pp. 201–30 (1991).

8 Jo, H., Song, C. & Miyazaki, Y., 'Physiological Benefits of Viewing Nature: A Systematic Review of Indoor Experiments', *International Journal of Environmental Research and Public Health* 16, 4,739 (2019).

9 Stevenson, M. P., Schilhab, T. & Bentsen, P., 'Attention Restoration Theory II: a systematic review to clarify attention processes affected by exposure to natural environments', *Journal of Toxicology and Environmental Health, Part B* 21, pp. 227–68, doi:10.1080/10937404.2018.1505571 (2018).

10 Dadvand, P. et al., 'Green spaces and cognitive development in primary schoolchildren', *Proceedings of the National Academy of Sciences* 112, pp. 7,937–42 (2015).

11 Lee, D., *Nature's Palette*, University of Chicago Press, Chicago, 2010.

12 Kaplan, R. & Kaplan, S., *The Experience of Nature: A Psychological Perspective*, Cambridge University Press, Cambridge, 1989; Kaplan, S., 'The restorative benefits of nature: Toward an integrative framework', Journal of Environmental Psychology 15, pp. 169–82 (1995).

13 Kaplan, S. & Berman, M. G., 'Directed attention as a common resource for executive functioning and self-regulation', *Perspectives on Psychological Science* 5, pp. 43–57 (2010).

14 Willis, K. & McElwain, J., *The Evolution of Plants*, Oxford University Press, Oxford, 2014.

15 Orians, G., Heerwagen, J., Barkow, J., Cosmides, L. & Tooby, J., 'The adapted mind: Evolutionary psychology and the generation of culture', *The Adapted Mind: Evolutionary Psychology and the Generation of Culture*, Oxford University Press, Oxford, pp. 555–79 (1992).

16 Summit, J. & Sommer, R., 'Further studies of preferred tree shapes', *Environment and Behavior* 31, pp. 550–76 (1999).

17 Gerstenberg, T. & Hofmann, M., 'Perception and preference of trees: A psychological contribution to tree species selection in urban areas', *Urban Forestry & Urban Greening* 15, pp. 103–11 (2016).

18 Balling, J. D. & Falk, J. H., 'Development of visual preference for natural environments', *Environment and Behavior* 14, pp. 5–28 (1982).

19 Hägerhäll, C. M., 'Responses to nature from populations of varied cultural background', in Bosch, M. and Bird, W. (eds), *Oxford Textbook of Nature and Public Health*, Oxford University Press, Oxford, 2018.

20 Falk, J. H. & Balling, J. D., 'Evolutionary influence on human landscape preference', *Environment and Behavior* 42, pp. 479–93 (2010).

21 Hägerhäll, C. M. et al., 'Do humans really prefer semi-open natural landscapes? A cross-cultural reappraisal', *Frontiers in Psychology* 9, p. 822 (2018); Moura, J. M. B., Ferreira Júnior, W. S., Silva, T. C. & Albuquerque, U. P., 'The Influence of the Evolutionary Past on the Mind: An Analysis of the Preference

for Landscapes in the Human Species', *Frontiers in Psychology* 9, 2,485, doi:10.3389/fpsyg.2018.02485 (2018).

22   Hägerhäll, C. M. et al., 'Investigations of human EEG response to viewing fractal patterns', *Perception* 37, pp. 1,488–94 (2008); Taylor, R. P., Spehar, B., Van Donkelaar, P. & Hagerhall, C. M., 'Perceptual and physiological responses to Jackson Pollock's fractals', *Frontiers in Human Neuroscience* 5, p. 60 (2011); Taylor, R. P., 'Reduction of physiological stress using fractal art and architecture', *Leonardo* 39, pp. 245–51 (2006).

23   Mandelbrot, B. B., *The Fractal Geometry of Nature*, W. H. Freeman and Company, New York, 8, p. 406 (1983).

24   Taylor et al., 'Perceptual and physiological responses to Jackson Pollock's fractals'.

25   Taylor, 'Reduction of physiological stress using fractal art and architecture'.

26   Hägerhäll, C. M., Purcell, T. & Taylor, R., 'Fractal dimension of landscape silhouette outlines as a predictor of landscape preference', *Journal of Environmental Psychology* 24, pp. 247–55 (2004).

27   Hägerhäll, 'Investigations of human EEG response to viewing fractal patterns'.

28   Van den Berg, A. E., Joye, Y. & Koole, S. L., 'Why viewing nature is more fascinating and restorative than viewing buildings: A closer look at perceived complexity', *Urban Forestry & Urban Greening* 20, pp. 397–401 (2016).

29   Ho, S., Mohtadi, A., Daud, K., Leonards, U. & Handy, T. C., 'Using smartphone accelerometry to assess the relationship between cognitive load and gait dynamics during outdoor walking', *Scientific Reports* 9, pp. 1–13 (2019).

30   Jiang, B., Chang, C.-Y. & Sullivan, W. C., 'A dose of nature: Tree cover, stress reduction, and gender differences', *Landscape and Urban Planning* 132, pp. 26–36 (2014).

2 WHY GREEN IS GOOD FOR US, AND NOT JUST
IN WHAT WE EAT

1   Thoreau, H.D.W., *Walden, or Life in the Woods*, Ticknor and Fields, Boston, 1854.

2   Kaufman, A. J. & Lohr, V. I., in *VIII International People–Plant Symposium on Exploring Therapeutic Powers of Flowers, Greenery and Nature* 790, pp. 179–84; Lohr, V. I., 'Benefits of nature: what we are learning about why people respond to nature', Journal of Physiological Anthropology 26, pp. 83–5 (2007).

3   Lee, *Nature's Palette.*

4   Glover, B. J. & Whitney, H. M., 'Structural colour and iridescence in plants: the poorly studied relations of pigment colour', *Annals of Botany* 105, pp. 505–11 (2010).

5   Airoldi, C. A., Ferria, J. & Glover, B. J., 'The cellular and genetic basis of structural colour in plants', *Current Opinion in Plant Biology* 47, pp. 81–7 (2019).

6   Lichtenfeld, S., Elliot, A. J., Maier, M. A. & Pekrun, R., 'Fertile green: Green facilitates creative performance', *Personality and Social Psychology Bulletin* 38, pp. 784–97 (2012).

7   Akers, A. et al., 'Visual color perception in green exercise: Positive effects on mood and perceived exertion', *Environmental Science & Technology* 46, pp. 8,661–6 (2012).

8   Poldrack, R. A., *The New Mind Readers: What neuroimaging can and cannot reveal about our thoughts*, Princeton University Press, Princeton, 2018.

9   Racey, C., Franklin, A. & Bird, C. M., 'The processing of color preference in the brain', *Neuroimage* 191, pp. 529–36 (2019).

10   Ibid.

11   Elsadek, M., Sun, M. & Fujii, E., 'Psycho-physiological responses to plant variegation as measured through eye movement, self-reported emotion and cerebral activity', *Indoor and Built Environment* 26, pp. 758–70 (2017).

12   Martinez-Conde, S., Macknik, S. L., Troncoso, X. G. & Hubel, D. H., 'Microsaccades: a neurophysiological analysis', *Trends in Neurosciences* 32, pp. 463–75 (2009).

13   McCamy, M. B., Otero-Millan, J., Di Stasi, L. L., Macknik, S. L. & Martinez-Conde, S., 'Highly informative natural scene regions increase microsaccade production during visual scanning', *Journal of Neuroscience* 34, pp. 2,956–66 (2014).

14   Elsadek et al., 'Psycho-physiological responses to plant variegation as measured through eye movement, self-reported emotion and cerebral activity'.

15 Kexiu, L., Elsadek, M., Liu, B. & Fujii, E., 'Foliage colors improve relaxation and emotional status of university students from different countries', *Heliyon* 7, e06131 (2021).

16 Archetti, M. et al., 'Unravelling the evolution of autumn colours: an interdisciplinary approach', *Trends in Ecology & Evolution* 24, pp. 166–73 (2009).

17 Schloss, K. B. & Heck, I. A., 'Seasonal changes in color preferences are linked to variations in environmental colors: a longitudinal study of fall', *I-Perception* 8, 2041669517742177 (2017).

18 Paddle, E. & Gilliland, J., 'Orange Is the New Green: Exploring the Restorative Capacity of Seasonal Foliage in Schoolyard Trees', *International Journal of Environmental Research and Public Health* 13, p. 497 (2016).

19 Paraskevopoulou, A. T. et al., 'The impact of seasonal colour change in planting on patients with psychotic disorders using biosensors', *Urban Forestry & Urban Greening* 36, pp. 50–6, doi:https://doi.org/10.1016/j.ufug.2018.09.006 (2018).

3 FLOWER POWER

1 Willis, K. et al., *State of the world's plants 2017*, Royal Botanic Gardens Kew, London, 2017.

2 Morton, J. W., *250 Beautiful Flowers and How to Grow Them*, Foulsham, London, 1939.

3 Haviland-Jones, J., Rosario, H. H., Wilson, P. & McGuire, T. R., 'An Environmental Approach to Positive Emotion: Flowers', *Evolutionary Psychology* 3, 147470490500300109, doi:10.1177/147470490500300109 (2005).

4 Ikei, H., Komatsu, M., Song, C., Himoro, E. & Miyazaki, Y., 'The physiological and psychological relaxing effects of viewing rose flowers in office workers', *Journal of Physiological Anthropology* 33, 6, doi:10.1186/1880-6805-33-6 (2014).

5 Ibid.

6 Willis & McElwain, *The Evolution of Plants*.

7 Glover, B., *Understanding Flowers and Flowering*, Oxford University Press, Oxford, 2014 (2nd ed.).

8 Lee, *Nature's Palette*.

9   Glover, *Understanding Flowers and Flowering*.
10 Whitney, H. M. et al., 'Floral Iridescence, Produced by Diffractive Optics, Acts as a Cue for Animal Pollinators', *Science* 323, pp. 130–3 (2009).
11 Vignolini, S. et al., 'Directional scattering from the glossy flower of Ranunculus: how the buttercup lights up your chin', *Journal of the Royal Society Interface* 9, 1,295–301, doi:10.1098/rsif.2011.0759 (2012).
12 Yue, C. & Behe, B. K., 'Consumer Color Preferences for Single-stem Cut Flowers on Calendar Holidays and Noncalendar Occasions', *HortScience* 45, 78–82, doi:10.21273/hortsci.45.1.78 (2010).
13 Ibid.
14 Hula, M. & Flegr, J., 'What flowers do we like? The influence of shape and color on the rating of flower beauty', *PeerJ* 4, e2106, doi:10.7717/peerj.2106 (2016).
15 Willis, K., *Plants: From Roots to Riches*, Hachette, London, 2014.
16 Jang, H. S., Kim, J., Kim, K. S. & Pak, C. H., 'Human brain activity and emotional responses to plant color stimuli', *Color Research & Application* 39, pp. 307–16 (2014).
17 Xie, J., Liu, B. & Elsadek, M., 'How Can Flowers and Their Colors Promote Individuals' Physiological and Psychological States during the COVID-19 Lockdown?', *International Journal of Environmental Research and Public Health* 18, 10,258 (2021).
18 Jang et al., 'Human brain activity and emotional responses to plant color stimuli'.
19 Xie et al., 'How Can Flowers and Their Colors Promote Individuals' Physiological and Psychological States during the COVID-19 Lockdown?'.
20 Singh, S., *https://www.marketresearchfuture.com/reports/artificial-plants-market-10585*, (2023).
21 Igarashi, M., Aga, M., Ikei, H., Namekawa, T. & Miyazaki, Y., 'Physiological and Psychological Effects on High School Students of Viewing Real and Artificial Pansies', *International Journal of Environmental Research and Public Health* 12, pp. 2,521–31 (2015).
22 Hoyle, H., Hitchmough, J. & Jorgensen, A., 'All about the "wow factor"? The relationships between aesthetics, restorative

effect and perceived biodiversity in designed urban planting', *Landscape and Urban Planning* 164, pp. 109–23, doi:https://doi. org/10.1016/j.landurbplan.2017.03.011 (2017).

23 Graves, R. A., Pearson, S. M. & Turner, M. G., 'Species richness alone does not predict cultural ecosystem service value', *Proceedings of the National Academy of Sciences* 114, pp. 3,774–9, doi:10.1073/pnas.1701370114 (2017).

24 Wang, R., Zhao, J., Meitner, M. J., Hu, Y. & Xu, X., 'Characteristics of urban green spaces in relation to aesthetic preference and stress recovery', *Urban Forestry & Urban Greening* 41, pp. 6–13, doi:https://doi.org/10.1016/j.ufug.2019.03.005 (2019).

25 Jiang, Y. & Yuan, T., 'Public perceptions and preferences for wildflower meadows in Beijing, China', *Urban Forestry & Urban Greening* 27, pp. 324–31, doi:https://doi.org/10.1016/j. ufug.2017.07.004 (2017).

4 THE SWEET SMELL OF SUCCESS

1 Littman, R. J., Silverstein, J., Goldsmith, D., Coughlin, S. & Mashaly, H., 'Eau de Cleopatra: Mendesian Perfume and Tell Timai', *Near Eastern Archaeology* 84, pp. 216–29 (2021).

2 Kemp, S., 'A medieval controversy about odor', *Journal of the History of the Behavioral Sciences* 33, pp. 211–19 (1997).

3 Ibid.

4 Wåhlin, A., *Dissertatio medica odores medicamentorum exhibens*, Vol. 1, Typis Laurentii Salvii, 1752.

5 Ibid.

6 Barwich, A.-S., *Smellosophy*, Harvard University Press, Harvard, 2020.

7 Bushdid, C., Magnasco, M. O., Vosshall, L. B. & Keller, A., 'Humans can discriminate more than 1 trillion olfactory stimuli', *Science* 343, pp. 1370–2 (2014).

8 Barwich, *Smellosophy*.

9 Sowndhararajan, K. & Kim, S., 'Influence of fragrances on human psychophysiological activity: With special reference to human electroencephalographic response', *Scientia pharmaceutica* 84, pp. 724–51 (2016).

10 Sumitomo, K. et al., 'Conifer-derived monoterpenes and forest walking', *Mass Spectrometry* 4, A0042–A0042 (2015).

11 Sowndhararajan & Kim, 'Influence of fragrances on human psychophysiological activity'.

12 McGee, H., *Nose Dive: A Field Guide to the World's Smells*, Hachette, London, 2020.

13 Ibid.

14 Andersen, L., Corazon, S.S.S. & Stigsdotter, U.K.K., 'Nature exposure and its effects on immune system functioning: a systematic review', *International Journal of Environmental Research and Public Health* 18, 1,416 (2021).

15 Willis & McElwain, *The Evolution of Plants*.

16 Ibid.

17 Wen, Y., Yan, Q., Pan, Y., Gu, X. & Liu, Y., 'Medical empirical research on forest bathing (Shinrin-yoku): A systematic review', *Environmental Health and Preventive Medicine* 24, pp. 1–21 (2019).

18 Ibid.

19 Miyazaki, *Shinrin Yoku: The Japanese Art of Forest Bathing*.

20 Ikei, H., Song, C. & Miyazaki, Y., 'Effects of olfactory stimulation by α-pinene on autonomic nervous activity', *Journal of Wood Science* 62, pp. 568–72 (2016).

21 Kim, J.-C. et al., 'The potential benefits of therapeutic treatment using gaseous terpenes at ambient low levels', *Applied Sciences* 9, 4,507 (2019).

22 Tsunetsugu, Y. & Ishibashi, K., 'Heart rate and heart rate variability in infants during olfactory stimulation', *Annals of Human Biology* 46, pp. 347–53 (2019).

23 Ibid.

24 Ikei, H., Song, C. & Miyazaki, Y., 'Physiological effect of olfactory stimulation by Hinoki cypress (Chamaecyparis obtusa) leaf oil', *Journal of Physiological Anthropology* 34, pp. 1–7 (2015).

25 Li, Q. et al., 'Effect of phytoncide from trees on human natural killer cell function', *International Journal of Immunopathology and Pharmacology* 22, pp. 951–9 (2009).

26 Tsao, T.-M. et al., 'Health effects of a forest environment on natural killer cells in humans: An observational pilot study', *Oncotarget* 9, 16,501 (2018).

t /

27 Li, Q., 'Effect of forest bathing trips on human immune function', *Environmental Health and Preventive Medicine* 15, pp. 9–17 (2010); Li, Q. et al., 'A forest bathing trip increases human natural killer activity and expression of anti-cancer proteins in female subjects', *Journal of Biological Regulators and Homeostatic Agents* 22, pp. 45–55 (2008).

28 Wu, G. A. et al., 'Genomics of the origin and evolution of Citrus', *Nature* 554, pp. 311–16 (2018).

29 Christenhusz, M. J., Fay, M. F. & Chase, M. W., in *Plants of the World*, University of Chicago Press, Chicago, 2017.

30 Cho, K. S. et al., 'Terpenes from forests and human health', *Toxicological Research* 33, pp. 97–106 (2017).

31 Vieira, A. J., Beserra, F. P., Souza, M., Totti, B. & Rozza, A., 'Limonene: Aroma of innovation in health and disease', *Chemico-Biological Interactions* 283, pp. 97–106 (2018).

32 Ibid.

33 Aprotosoaie, A. C., Hǎncianu, M., Costache, I. I. & Miron, A., 'Linalool: a review on a key odorant molecule with valuable biological properties', *Flavour and Fragrance Journal* 29, pp. 193–219 (2014).

34 Ko, L.-W., Su, C.-H., Yang, M.-H., Liu, S.-Y. & Su, T.-P., 'A pilot study on essential oil aroma stimulation for enhancing slow-wave EEG in sleeping brain', *Scientific Reports* 11, 1078, doi:10.1038/s41598-020-80171-x (2021).

35 Donelli, D., Antonelli, M., Bellinazzi, C., Gensini, G. F. & Firenzuoli, F., 'Effects of lavender on anxiety: A systematic review and meta-analysis', *Phytomedicine* 65, 153099 (2019).

36 Ibid.

37 Harada, H., Kashiwadani, H., Kanmura, Y. & Kuwaki, T., 'Linalool Odor-Induced Anxiolytic Effects in Mice', *Frontiers in Behavioral Neuroscience* 12, doi:10.3389/fnbeh.2018.00241 (2018).

38 Ko et al., 'A pilot study on essential oil aroma stimulation for enhancing slow-wave EEG in sleeping brain'.

39 Diego, M. A. et al., 'Aromatherapy positively affects mood, EEG patterns of alertness and math computations', *International Journal of Neuroscience* 96, pp. 217–24 (1998).

40 Tschiggerl, C. & Bucar, F., 'Investigation of the volatile fraction of rosemary infusion extracts', *Scientia Pharmaceutica* 78, pp. 483–92 (2010); Sayorwan, W. et al., 'Effects of inhaled rosemary oil on subjective feelings and activities of the nervous system', *Scientia Pharmaceutica* 81, pp. 531–42 (2013).

41 Faridzadeh, A. et al., 'Neuroprotective Potential of Aromatic Herbs: Rosemary, Sage, and Lavender', *Frontiers in Neuroscience* 16, doi:10.3389/fnins.2022.909833 (2022).

42 Nasiri, A. & Boroomand, M. M., 'The effect of rosemary essential oil inhalation on sleepiness and alertness of shift-working nurses: A randomized, controlled field trial', *Complementary Therapies in Clinical Practice* 43, 101326 (2021).

43 Moss, M. & Oliver, L., 'Plasma 1, 8-cineole correlates with cognitive performance following exposure to rosemary essential oil aroma', *Therapeutic Advances in Psychopharmacology* 2, pp. 103–13 (2012).

44 Hoult, L., Longstaff, L. & Moss, M., 'Prolonged low-level exposure to the aroma of peppermint essential oil enhances aspects of cognition and mood in healthy adults', *American Journal of Plant Sciences* 10, pp. 1,002–12 (2019).

45 Fang, R., Zweig, M., Li, J., Mirzababaei, J. & Simmonds, M. S., 'Diversity of volatile organic compounds in 14 rose cultivars', *Journal of Essential Oil Research* 35, pp. 220–37 (2023).

46 McGee, *Nose Dive*.

47 Caser, M. & Scariot, V., 'The Contribution of Volatile Organic Compounds (VOCs) Emitted by Petals and Pollen to the Scent of Garden Roses', *Horticulturae* 8, 1049 (2022).

48 Igarashi, M., Song, C., Ikei, H., Ohira, T. & Miyazaki, Y., 'Effect of olfactory stimulation by fresh rose flowers on autonomic nervous activity', *Journal of Alternative and Complementary Medicine* 20, pp. 727–31, doi:10.1089/acm.2014.0029 (2014).

49 Dmitrenko, D. et al., 'Caroma Therapy: Pleasant Scents Promote Safer Driving, Better Mood, and Improved Wellbeing in Angry Drivers' in *Proceedings of the 2020 Chi Conference on Human Factors in Computing Systems*, pp. 1–13.

50 Ibid.

5 SOUND SURGERY

1 Morillas, J.M.B., Gozalo, G. R.,González, D. M., Moraga, P. A. & Vílchez-Gómez, R., 'Noise pollution and urban planning', *Current Pollution Reports* 4, pp. 208–19 (2018).

2 World Health Organization, *Environmental noise guidelines for the European region* (2018).

3 Hedblom, M., Knez, I., Ode Sang, Å. & Gunnarsson, B., 'Evaluation of natural sounds in urban greenery: potential impact for urban nature preservation', *Royal Society Open Science* 4, 170037 (2017).

4 Krzywicka, P. & Byrka, K., 'Restorative qualities of and preference for natural and urban soundscapes', *Frontiers in Psychology* 8, 1705 (2017).

5 Ratcliffe, E., 'Sound and soundscape in restorative natural environments: A narrative literature review', *Frontiers in Psychology* 12, 963 (2021).

6 Ratcliffe, E., Gatersleben, B. & Sowden, P. T., 'Bird sounds and their contributions to perceived attention restoration and stress recovery', *Journal of Environmental Psychology* 36, pp. 221–8 (2013).

7 Bjork, E., 'The perceived quality of natural sounds', *Acustica* 58, pp. 185-8 (1985); Zhao, W., Li, H., Zhu, X. & Ge, T., 'Effect of birdsong soundscape on perceived restorativeness in an urban park', *International Journal of Environmental Research and Public Health* 17, 5659 (2020).

8 Merlin (app) available at <https://merlin.allaboutbirds.org> (2023).

9 Ratcliffe, E., Gatersleben, B. & Sowden, P. T., 'Predicting the perceived restorative potential of bird sounds through acoustics and aesthetics', *Environment and Behavior* 52, pp. 371–400 (2020).

10 Ratcliffe, E., Gatersleben, B. & Sowden, P. T., 'Associations with bird sounds: How do they relate to perceived restorative potential?' *Journal of Environmental Psychology* 47, pp. 136–44, doi:https://doi.org/10.1016/j.jenvp.2016.05.009 (2016).

11   Ratcliffe et al., 'Predicting the perceived restorative potential of bird sounds through acoustics and aesthetics'.

12   Jo, H. et al., 'Physiological and psychological effects of forest and urban sounds using high-resolution sound sources', *International Journal of Environmental Research and Public Health* 16, 2649 (2019).

13   Li, Z. & Kang, J., 'Sensitivity analysis of changes in human physiological indicators observed in soundscapes', *Landscape and Urban Planning* 190, 103593 (2019).

14   Kaplan, S., 'The restorative benefits of nature: Toward an integrative framework', *Journal of Environmental Psychology* 15, pp. 169–82 (1995).

15   Van Hedger, S. C. et al., 'Of cricket chirps and car horns: The effect of nature sounds on cognitive performance', *Psychonomic Bulletin & Review* 26, pp. 522–30, doi:10.3758/s13423-018-1539-1 (2019).

16   Arai, Y. C. et al., 'Intra-operative natural sound decreases salivary amylase activity of patients undergoing inguinal hernia repair under epidural anesthesia', *Acta Anaesthesiologica Scandinavica* 52, pp. 987–90 (2008).

17   Saadatmand, V. et al., 'Effects of natural sounds on pain: A randomized controlled trial with patients receiving mechanical ventilation support', *Pain Management Nursing* 16, pp. 483–92 (2015).

18   Farzaneh, M. et al., 'Comparative effect of nature-based sounds intervention and headphones intervention on pain severity after cesarean section: A prospective double-blind randomized trial', *Anesthesiology and Pain Medicine* 9 (2019).

19   Buxton, R. T., Pearson, A. L., Allou, C., Fristrup, K. & Wittemyer, G., 'A synthesis of health benefits of natural sounds and their distribution in national parks', *Proceedings of the National Academy of Sciences* 118, e2013097118 (2021).

20   Ibid.

21   Annerstedt, M. et al., 'Inducing physiological stress recovery with sounds of nature in a virtual reality forest – Results from a pilot study', *Physiology & Behavior* 118, pp. 240–50 (2013).

22   Ibid.

23 Hedblom, M. et al., 'Reduction of physiological stress by urban green space in a multisensory virtual experiment', *Scientific Reports* 9, pp. 1–11 (2019).

24 Ibid.

25 Buxton et al., 'A synthesis of health benefits of natural sounds and their distribution in national parks'.

26 Uebel, K., Marselle, M., Dean, A. J., Rhodes, J. R. & Bonn, A., 'Urban green space soundscapes and their perceived restorativeness', *People and Nature* 3, pp. 756–69 (2021).

27 Kogan, P., Gale, T., Arenas, J. P. & Arias, C., 'Development and application of practical criteria for the recognition of potential Health Restoration Soundscapes (HeReS) in urban greenspaces', *Science of The Total Environment* 793, 148541 (2021).

6 THE PROVEN HEALTH BENEFITS OF TREE-HUGGING

1 Crossman, M. K., Kazdin, A. E., Matijczak, A., Kitt, E. R. & Santos, L. R., 'The influence of interactions with dogs on affect, anxiety, and arousal in children', *Journal of Clinical Child & Adolescent Psychology* 49, pp. 535–48 (2020).

2 Cipriani, J. et al., 'A systematic review of the effects of horticultural therapy on persons with mental health conditions', *Occupational Therapy in Mental Health* 33, pp. 47–69 (2017); Han, A.-R., Park, S.-A. & Ahn, B.-E., 'Reduced stress and improved physical functional ability in elderly with mental health problems following a horticultural therapy program', *Complementary Therapies in Medicine* 38, pp. 19–23 (2018).

3 Oh, Y.-A., Park, S.-A. & Ahn, B.-E., 'Assessment of the psychopathological effects of a horticultural therapy program in patients with schizophrenia', *Complementary Therapies in Medicine* 36, pp. 54–8 (2018); Scartazza, A. et al., 'Caring local biodiversity in a healing garden: Therapeutic benefits in young subjects with autism', *Urban Forestry & Urban Greening* 47, 126511 (2020).

4 Koga, K. & Iwasaki, Y., 'Psychological and physiological effect in humans of touching plant foliage – using the semantic differential method and cerebral activity as indicators', *Journal of Physiological Anthropology* 32, pp. 1–9 (2013).

5   Sakuragawa, S., Kaneko, T. & Miyazaki, Y., 'Effects of contact with wood on blood pressure and subjective evaluation', *Journal of Wood Science* 54, pp. 107–13 (2008).

6   Ikei, H., Song, C. & Miyazaki, Y., 'Physiological effects of touching wood', *International Journal of Environmental Research and Public Health* 14, 801 (2017).

7   Ibid.

8   Ikei, H., Song, C. & Miyazaki, Y., 'Physiological effects of touching the wood of hinoki cypress (Chamaecyparis obtusa) with the soles of the feet', *International Journal of Environmental Research and Public Health* 15, 2135 (2018).

9   Bhatta, S. R., Tiippana, K., Vahtikari, K., Hughes, M. & Kyttä, M., 'Sensory and emotional perception of wooden surfaces through fingertip touch', *Frontiers in Psychology* 8, 367 (2017).

10 Ibid.

11 Sakuragawa et al., 'Effects of contact with wood on blood pressure and subjective evaluation'.

12 Shao, Y., Elsadek, M. & Liu, B., 'Horticultural activity: Its contribution to stress recovery and wellbeing for children', *International Journal of Environmental Research and Public Health* 17, 1229 (2020).

13 Ibid.

14 Kim, S.-O., Jeong, J.-E., Oh, Y.-A., Kim, H.-R. & Park, S.-A., 'Comparing concentration levels and emotional states of children using electroencephalography during horticultural and nonhorticultural activities', *HortScience* 56, pp. 324–9 (2021).

15 Ibid.

16 Hutmacher, F., 'Why is there so much more research on vision than on any other sensory modality?', *Frontiers in Psychology* 10, 2246 (2019).

17 Ibid.

18 Ibid.

19 Xu, Y. et al., 'Mitochondrial function modulates touch signalling in Arabidopsis thaliana', *The Plant Journal* 97, pp. 623–45 (2019).

7 HIDDEN SENSES

1   Roslund, M. I. et al., 'Biodiversity intervention enhances immune regulation and health-associated commensal microbiota among daycare children', *Science Advances* 6, eaba2578 (2020).

2   Rinninella, E. et al., 'What is the healthy gut microbiota composition? A changing ecosystem across age, environment, diet, and diseases', *Microorganisms* 7, 14 (2019).

3   Roslund et al., 'Biodiversity intervention enhances immune regulation and health-associated commensal microbiota among daycare children'.

4   Rinninella et al., 'What is the healthy gut microbiota composition? A changing ecosystem across age, environment, diet, and diseases'.

5   Avery, E. G. et al., 'The gut microbiome in hypertension: recent advances and future perspectives', *Circulation Research* 128, pp. 934–50 (2021).

6   Hirt, H., 'Healthy soils for healthy plants for healthy humans: How beneficial microbes in the soil, food and gut are interconnected and how agriculture can contribute to human health', *EMBO Reports* 21, e51069 (2020).

7   Enders, G., *Gut: The Inside Story of Our Body's Most Underrated Organ (Revised Edition)*, Greystone Books, New York, 2018.

8   Hirt, 'Healthy soils for healthy plants for healthy humans'.

9   Rinninella, 'What is the healthy gut microbiota composition? A changing ecosystem across age, environment, diet, and diseases'; Avery, E. G. et al., 'The gut microbiome in hypertension: recent advances and future perspectives', *Circulation Research* 128, pp. 934–50 (2021).

10 Rothschild, D. et al., 'Environment dominates over host genetics in shaping human gut microbiota', *Nature* 555, pp. 210–15 (2018).

11 Blum, H. E., 'The human microbiome', *Advances in Medical Sciences* 62, pp. 414–20 (2017).

12 Enders, *Gut*.

13 Hitch, T. C. et al., 'Microbiome-based interventions to modulate gut ecology and the immune system', *Mucosal Immunology* 15, pp. 1,095–113 (2022).

14 Hirt, 'Healthy soils for healthy plants for healthy humans'.

15 Enders, *Gut*.

16 Flandroy, L. et al., 'The impact of human activities and lifestyles on the interlinked microbiota and health of humans and of ecosystems', *Science of The Total Environment* 627, pp. 1,018–38 (2018).

17 Von Hertzen, L., Hanski, I. & Haahtela, T., 'Natural immunity: biodiversity loss and inflammatory diseases are two global megatrends that might be related', *EMBO Reports* 12, pp. 1,089–93 (2011).

18 Rook, G. A., 'Regulation of the immune system by biodiversity from the natural environment: an ecosystem service essential to health', *Proceedings of the National Academy of Sciences* 110, pp. 18,360–7 (2013).

19 Mhuireach, G. et al., 'Urban greenness influences airborne bacterial community composition', *Science of The Total Environment* 571, pp. 680–7 (2016); Mills, J. G. et al., 'Urban habitat restoration provides a human health benefit through microbiome rewilding: the Microbiome Rewilding Hypothesis', *Restoration Ecology* 25, pp. 866–72 (2017); Selway, C. A. et al., 'Transfer of environmental microbes to the skin and respiratory tract of humans after urban green space exposure', *Environment International* 145, 106084 (2020); Nielsen, C. C. et al., 'Natural environments in the urban context and gut microbiota in infants', *Environment International* 142, 105881 (2020).

20 Mahnert, A., Moissl-Eichinger, C. & Berg, G., 'Microbiome interplay: plants alter microbial abundance and diversity within the built environment', *Frontiers in Microbiology* 6, 887 (2015).

21 Hanski, I. et al., 'Environmental biodiversity, human microbiota, and allergy are interrelated', *Proceedings of the National Academy of Sciences* 109, pp. 8,334–9 (2012).

22 Parajuli, A. et al., 'Yard vegetation is associated with gut microbiota composition', *Science of The Total Environment* 713, 136707 (2020).

23 Grönroos, M. et al., 'Short-term direct contact with soil and plant materials leads to an immediate increase in diversity of skin microbiota', *MicrobiologyOpen* 8, e00645 (2019).

24 Selway et al., 'Transfer of environmental microbes to the skin and respiratory tract of humans after urban green space exposure'.

25 Tischer, C. et al., 'Interplay between natural environment, human microbiota and immune system: A scoping review of interventions and future perspectives towards allergy prevention', *Science of The Total Environment*, 153422 (2022).

26 Hanski et al., 'Environmental biodiversity, human microbiota, and allergy are interrelated'.

27 Parajuli et al., 'Yard vegetation is associated with gut microbiota composition'.

28 Tischer et al., 'Interplay between natural environment, human microbiota and immune system'.

29 Roslund, M. I. et al., 'A Placebo-controlled double-blinded test of the biodiversity hypothesis of immune-mediated diseases: Environmental microbial diversity elicits changes in cytokines and increase in T regulatory cells in young children', *Ecotoxicology and Environmental Safety* 242, 113900 (2022).

30 Nurminen, N. et al., 'Nature-derived microbiota exposure as a novel immunomodulatory approach', *Future Microbiology* 13, pp. 737–44 (2018).

31 Blum, H. E., 'The human microbiome', *Advances in Medical Sciences* 62, pp. 414–20 (2017).

32 Grönroos et al., 'Short-term direct contact with soil and plant materials leads to an immediate increase in diversity of skin microbiota'.

8 INDOOR SENSESCAPES

1 Redlich, C. A., Sparer, J. & Cullen, M. R., 'Sick-building syndrome', *The Lancet* 349, pp. 1,013–16 (1997).

2   Ghaffarianhoseini, A. et al., 'Sick building syndrome: are we doing enough?', *Architectural Science Review* 61, pp. 99–121 (2018).

3   Kellert, S. R., *Nature by Design: The practice of biophilic design*, Yale University Press, Yale, 2018.

4   Willis, *Plants: From Roots to Riches*.

5   Plat, H., *Floraes Paradise*, London, 1608.

6   Horwood, C., *Potted History: The Story of Plants in the Home*, Frances Lincoln, London, 2007.

7   Maunder, M., *House Plants*, Reaktion Books, London, 2022.

8   Ibid.

9   Kellert, *Nature by Design*.

10 Wilson, *Biophilia*.

11 Kellert, *Nature by Design*.

12 Gillis, K. & Gatersleben, B., 'A review of psychological literature on the health and wellbeing benefits of biophilic design', *Buildings* 5, pp. 948–63 (2015).

13 Han, K.-T. & Ruan, L.-W., 'Effects of indoor plants on air quality: a systematic review', *Environmental Science and Pollution Research* 27, pp. 16,019–51, doi:10.1007/s11356-020-08174-9 (2020).

14 United Nations Environment Programme, *Pollution Action Note – Data you need to know*, https://www.unep.org/interactive/air-pollution-note/?gclid=CjwKCAjwue6hBhBVEiwA9YTx8Bi4oAvpuLmcPXaLm2aqJCrXIylT3uWCfaQAjc4k92EMHnnyHgKKWxoC_wMQAvD_BwE (2022).

15 Matheson, S., Fleck, R., Irga, P. & Torpy, F., 'Phytoremediation for the indoor environment: a state-of-the-art review', *Reviews in Environmental Science and Bio/Technology*, pp. 1–32 (2023).

16 Wolverton, B. C., Douglas, W. L. & Bounds, K., 'A study of interior landscape plants for indoor air pollution abatement', NASA Technical Reports Server, 1989.

17 Pettit, T., Irga, P. & Torpy, F., 'The in situ pilot-scale phytoremediation of airborne VOCs and particulate matter with an active green wall', *Air Quality, Atmosphere & Health* 12, pp. 33–44 (2019).

18 Ibid.

19 Jo, H., Song, C. & Miyazaki, Y., 'Physiological Benefits of Viewing Nature: A Systematic Review of Indoor Experiments', *International Journal of Environmental Research and Public Health* 16, 4739 (2019).

20 Van den Berg, A. E., Wesselius, J. E., Maas, J. & Tanja-Dijkstra, K., 'Green walls for a restorative classroom environment: a controlled evaluation study', *Environment and Behavior* 49, pp. 791–813 (2017).

21 Ibid.

22 Soininen, L. et al., 'Indoor green wall affects health-associated commensal skin microbiota and enhances immune regulation: a randomized trial among urban office workers', *Scientific Reports* 12, pp. 1–9 (2022).

23 Alapieti, T., Mikkola, R., Pasanen, P. & Salonen, H., 'The influence of wooden interior materials on indoor environment: a review', *European Journal of Wood and Wood Products* 78, pp. 617–34 (2020); Zhang, X., Lian, Z. & Wu, Y., 'Human physiological responses to wooden indoor environment', *Physiology & Behavior* 174, pp. 27–34 (2017); Shen, J., Zhang, X. & Lian, Z., 'Impact of wooden versus nonwooden interior designs on office workers' cognitive performance', *Perceptual and Motor Skills* 127, pp. 36–51 (2020).

24 Pohleven, J., Burnard, M. D. & Kutnar, A., 'Volatile organic compounds emitted from untreated and thermally modified wood-a review', *Wood and Fiber Science* 51, pp. 231–54 (2019).

25 Ibid.

26 Matsubara, E. & Kawai, S., 'VOCs emitted from Japanese cedar (Cryptomeria japonica) interior walls induce physiological relaxation', *Building and Environment* 72, pp. 125–30 (2014).

27 Jalilzadehazhari, E. & Johansson, J., 'Material properties of wooden surfaces used in interiors and sensory stimulation', *Wood Material Science & Engineering* (2019).

28 Nakamura, M., Ikei, H. & Miyazaki, Y., 'Physiological effects of visual stimulation with full-scale wall images composed of vertically and horizontally arranged wooden elements', *Journal of Wood Science* 65, pp. 1–11 (2019).

29 Shen, J., Zhang, X. & Lian, Z., 'Impact of wooden versus nonwooden interior designs on office workers' cognitive performance', *Perceptual and Motor Skills* 127, pp. 36–51 (2020).

30 Hirata, S., Toyoda, H. & Ohta, M., 'Reducing eye fatigue through the use of wood', *Journal of Wood Science* 63, pp. 401–8 (2017).

31 Burnard, M. D. & Kutnar, A., 'Human stress responses in office-like environments with wood furniture', *Building Research & Information* 48, pp. 316–30, doi:10.1080/09613218.2019.166060 9 (2020).

32 Kellert, *Nature by Design*.

33 Zhong, W., Schröder, T. & Bekkering, J., 'Biophilic design in architecture and its contributions to health, well-being, and sustainability: A critical review', *Frontiers of Architectural Research* 11, pp. 114–41, doi:https://doi.org/10.1016/j.foar.2021.07.006 (2022).

34 Gray, T. & Birrell, C., 'Are biophilic-designed site office buildings linked to health benefits and high performing occupants?', *International Journal of Environmental Research and Public Health* 11, pp. 12,204–22 (2014).

35 Yin, J. et al., 'Effects of biophilic interventions in office on stress reaction and cognitive function: A randomized crossover study in virtual reality', *Indoor Air* 29, pp. 1,028–39 (2019).

36 Yin, J. et al., 'Effects of biophilic indoor environment on stress and anxiety recovery: A between-subjects experiment in virtual reality', *Environment International* 136, 105427 (2020).

37 Yin et al., 'Effects of biophilic interventions in office on stress reaction and cognitive function'.

38 Aristizabal, S. et al., 'Biophilic office design: Exploring the impact of a multisensory approach on human well-being', *Journal of Environmental Psychology* 77, 101682 (2021).

39 Yin et al., 'Effects of biophilic indoor environment on stress and anxiety recovery'.

9 OUTDOOR SENSESCAPES

1 Twohig-Bennett, C. & Jones, A., 'The health benefits of the great outdoors: A systematic review and meta-analysis of

greenspace exposure and health outcomes', *Environmental Research* 166, pp. 628–37 (2018).

2 Song, C., Ikei, H., Igarashi, M., Takagaki, M. & Miyazaki, Y., 'Physiological and psychological effects of a walk in urban parks in fall', *International Journal of Environmental Research and Public Health* 12, pp. 14,216–28 (2015).

3 Bratman, G. N., Hamilton, J. P., Hahn, K. S., Daily, G. C. & Gross, J. J., 'Nature experience reduces rumination and subgenual prefrontal cortex activation', *Proceedings of the National Academy of Sciences* 112, pp. 8,567–72 (2015).

4 Ibid.

5 Taylor, H. A., 'Urban public parks, 1840–1900: design and meaning', *Garden History*, pp. 201–21 (1995).

6 Ibid.

7 Cranz, G., *The Politics of Park Design: A history of urban parks in America*, MIT Press, Boston, 1982.

8 Beil, K. & Hanes, D., 'The influence of urban natural and built environments on physiological and psychological measures of stress – A pilot study', *International Journal of Environmental Research and Public Health* 10, pp. 1,250–67 (2013).

9 Buxton et al., 'A synthesis of health benefits of natural sounds and their distribution in national parks'.

10 Gatersleben, B. & Andrews, M., 'When walking in nature is not restorative – The role of prospect and refuge', *Health & Place* 20, pp. 91–101 (2013).

11 Appleton, J., 'Prospects and refuges re-visited', *Landscape Journal* 3, pp. 91–103 (1984).

12 Gatersleben & Andrews, 'When walking in nature is not restorative – The role of prospect and refuge'.

13 Wang, R., Zhao, J., Meitner, M. J., Hu, Y. & Xu, X., 'Characteristics of urban green spaces in relation to aesthetic preference and stress recovery', *Urban Forestry & Urban Greening* 41, pp. 6–13, doi:https://doi.org/10.1016/j.ufug.2019.03.005 (2019).

14 Andersen, L., Corazon, S. S. S. & Stigsdotter, U. K. K., 'Nature exposure and its effects on immune system functioning: a systematic review', *International Journal of Environmental Research and Public Health* 18, 1416 (2021).

15 Robinson, J. M. et al., 'Exposure to airborne bacteria depends upon vertical stratification and vegetation complexity', *Scientific Reports* 11, 9516 (2021).

16 Mills, J. G. et al., 'Urban habitat restoration provides a human health benefit through microbiome rewilding: the Microbiome Rewilding Hypothesis', *Restoration Ecology* 25, pp. 866–72 (2017).

17 Hunter, M. R., Gillespie, B. W. & Chen, S. Y.-P., 'Urban nature experiences reduce stress in the context of daily life based on salivary biomarkers', *Frontiers in Psychology* 10, 722 (2019).

18 Ibid.

19 Wen, Y., Yan, Q., Pan, Y., Gu, X. & Liu, Y., 'Medical empirical research on forest bathing (Shinrin-yoku): A systematic review', *Environmental Health and Preventive Medicine* 24, pp. 1–21 (2019).

20 White, M. P. et al., 'Spending at least 120 minutes a week in nature is associated with good health and wellbeing', *Scientific Reports* 9, pp. 1–11 (2019).

21 Smith, J., 'Street Trees', via <https://www.buildingconservation.com/articles/street-trees/street-trees.htm> (2011).

22 Willis, K. J. & Petrokofsky, G., 'The natural capital of city trees', *Science* 356, pp. 374–6 (2017).

23 Eisenman, T. S. et al., 'Urban trees, air quality, and asthma: An interdisciplinary review', *Landscape and Urban Planning* 187, pp. 47–59, doi:https://doi.org/10.1016/j.landurbplan.2019.02.010 (2019).

24 Kardan, O. et al., 'Neighborhood greenspace and health in a large urban center', *Scientific Reports* 5, 11610, doi:10.1038/srep11610 (2015).

25 Ibid.

26 Taylor, M. S., Wheeler, B. W., White, M. P., Economou, T. & Osborne, N. J., 'Research note: Urban street tree density and antidepressant prescription rates – A cross-sectional study in London, UK', *Landscape and Urban Planning* 136, pp. 174–9 (2015).

27 Nguyen, P.-Y., Astell-Burt, T., Rahimi-Ardabili, H. & Feng, X., 'Green space quality and health: a systematic review',

International Journal of Environmental Research and Public Health 18, 11028 (2021).

28 Beil, K. & Hanes, D., 'The influence of urban natural and built environments on physiological and psychological measures of stress – A pilot study', *International Journal of Environmental Research and Public Health* 10, pp. 1,250–67 (2013).

29 Fonseca, F., Paschoalino, M. & Silva, L., 'Health and Well-Being Benefits of Outdoor and Indoor Vertical Greening Systems: A Review', *Sustainability* 15, 4107 (2023).

30 Vera, S., Viecco, M. & Jorquera, H., 'Effects of biodiversity in green roofs and walls on the capture of fine particulate matter', *Urban Forestry & Urban Greening* 63, 127229 (2021).

31 Fonseca, F., Paschoalino, M. & Silva, L., 'Health and Well-Being Benefits of Outdoor and Indoor Vertical Greening Systems: A Review', *Sustainability* 15, 4107 (2023).

32 Elsadek, M., Liu, B. & Lian, Z., 'Green façades: Their contribution to stress recovery and well-being in high-density cities', *Urban Forestry & Urban Greening* 46, 126446 (2019).

10 DIGGING FOR HEALTH

1 Statista, via <https://www.statista.com/statistics/1220222/global-gardening-sales-value/> (2022).

2 GfK, 'A quarter of the online population does gardening or yard work at least once a week', via <https://www.gfk.com/insights/a-quarter-of-the-online-population-does-gardening-or-yard-work-at-least-once-a-week> (2017).

3 Chalmin-Pui, L. S., Griffiths, A., Roe, J., Heaton, T. & Cameron, R., 'Why garden? – Attitudes and the perceived health benefits of home gardening', *Cities* 112, 103118 (2021).

4 Soga, M., Gaston, K. J. & Yamaura, Y., 'Gardening is beneficial for health: A meta-analysis', *Preventive Medicine Reports* 5, pp. 92–9 (2017).

5 Ibid.

6 Howarth, M., Brettle, A., Hardman, M. & Maden, M., 'What is the evidence for the impact of gardens and gardening on health and well-being: a scoping review and evidence-based logic model to guide healthcare strategy decision making on

the use of gardening approaches as a social prescription', *BMJ Open* 10, e036923 (2020).

7 Zhao, Y., Liu, Y. & Wang, Z., 'Effectiveness of horticultural therapy in people with dementia: A quantitative systematic review', *Journal of Clinical Nursing* 31, pp. 1983–97 (2022).

8 Lu, S., Zhao, Y., Liu, J., Xu, F. & Wang, Z., 'Effectiveness of horticultural therapy in people with schizophrenia: a systematic review and meta-analysis', *International Journal of Environmental Research and Public Health* 18, 964 (2021).

9 Hansen, M. M., Jones, R. & Tocchini, K., 'Shinrin-yoku (forest bathing) and nature therapy: A state-of-the-art review', *International Journal of Environmental Research and Public Health* 14, 851 (2017).

10 Ibid.

11 Howarth et al., 'What is the evidence for the impact of gardens and gardening on health and well-being'.

12 Haller, R. L., Kennedy, K. L. & Capra, C. L., *The Profession and Practice of Horticultural Therapy*, CRC Press, Florida, 2019.

13 American Horticultural Therapy Association, https://www.ahta.org (2020); THRIVE, The gardening for health charity <thrive.org.uk> (2023).

14 Stigsdotter, U. K. et al., 'Efficacy of nature-based therapy for individuals with stress-related illnesses: randomised controlled trial', *The British Journal of Psychiatry* 213, pp. 404–11 (2018).

15 Ibid.

16 Corazon, S. S., Nyed, P. K., Sidenius, U., Poulsen, D. V. & Stigsdotter, U. K., 'A long-term follow-up of the efficacy of nature-based therapy for adults suffering from stress-related illnesses on levels of healthcare consumption and sick-leave absence: a randomized controlled trial', *International Journal of Environmental Research and Public Health* 15, 137 (2018).

17 Stigsdotter et al., 'Efficacy of nature-based therapy for individuals with stress-related illnesses: randomised controlled trial'.

18 Busk, H. et al., 'Economic Evaluation of Nature-Based Therapy Interventions – A Scoping Review', *Challenges* 13, 23 (2022).

19 Pretty, J. & Barton, J., 'Nature-based interventions and mind–body interventions: Saving public health costs whilst

increasing life satisfaction and happiness', *International Journal of Environmental Research and Public Health* 17, 7769 (2020).

20 Ibid.

21 Reynolds, R., *On Guerrilla Gardening: A Handbook for Gardening without Boundaries*, Bloomsbury Publishing (London, 2014).

22 Chalmin – Pui, L. S. et al., '"It made me feel brighter in my-self"- The health and well-being impacts of a residential front garden horticultural intervention', *Landscape and Urban Planning* 205, 103958 (2021).

23 Ibid.

24 Young, C., Hofmann, M., Frey, D., Moretti, M. & Bauer, N., 'Psychological restoration in urban gardens related to garden type, biodiversity and garden-related stress', *Landscape and Urban Planning* 198, 103777 (2020).

25 Kaplan, S., 'The restorative benefits of nature: Toward an integrative framework', *Journal of Environmental Psychology* 15, pp. 169–82 (1995).

26 Hoyle et al., 'All about the "wow factor"?'.

27 Young et al., 'Psychological restoration in urban gardens related to garden type, biodiversity and garden-related stress'.

28 Spano, G. et al., 'Are community gardening and horticultural interventions beneficial for psychosocial well-being? A meta-analysis', *International Journal of Environmental Research and Public Health* 17, 3584 (2020).

29 Koay, W. I. & Dillon, D., 'Community gardening: Stress, well-being, and resilience potentials', *International Journal of Environmental Research and Public Health* 17, 6740 (2020).

30 Ibid.

31 Howarth et al., 'What is the evidence for the impact of gardens and gardening on health and well-being'.

32 Coventry, P. A. et al., 'Nature-based outdoor activities for mental and physical health: Systematic review and meta-analysis', *SSM-population Health* 16, 100934 (2021).

33 Ibid.

34 Thompson Coon, J. et al., 'Does participating in physical activity in outdoor natural environments have a greater effect on physical and mental wellbeing than physical activity indoors?

A systematic review', *Environmental Science & Technology* 45, pp. 1761–72 (2011).

35 Antonelli, M. et al., 'Forest volatile organic compounds and their effects on human health: A state-of-the-art review', *International Journal of Environmental Research and Public Health* 17, 6506 (2020).

PRESCRIBING NATURE

1 Grow to Know, via <https://www.growtoknow.co.uk> (2023).

2 Fyfe-Johnson, A. L. et al., 'Nature and children's health: a systematic review', *Pediatrics* 148 (2021).

3 Kondo, M. C. et al., 'Nature prescriptions for health: A review of evidence and research opportunities', *International Journal of Environmental Research and Public Health* 17, 4213 (2020); Dean, S., 'Seeing the Forest and the Trees: A Historical and Conceptual Look at Danish Forest Schools', *International Journal of Early Childhood Environmental Education* 6, pp. 53–63 (2019).

4 Nature Prescribed, via <https://parkrxamerica.org> (2023); Walk with a Doc, via <https://walkwithadoc.org> (2023); Fullam, J. et al., University of Exeter, Exeter, 2021; Association of Nature and Forest Therapy Programs, via <https://www.natureandforesttherapy.earth> (2023); Nature Prescribed, via <https://www.parkprescriptions.ca> (2023).

5 Markevych, I. et al., 'Exploring pathways linking greenspace to health: Theoretical and methodological guidance', *Environmental Research* 158, pp. 301–17 (2017).

6 Chang, M., Green, L. & Petrokofsky, C., *Public Health Spatial Planning in Practice: Improving Health and Wellbeing*, Policy Press, London, 2022.

7 Bratman, G. N. et al., 'Nature and mental health: An ecosystem service perspective', *Science Advances* 5, eaax0903 (2019).

Index

abutilon mosaic virus
  (*Begomovirus*), 71
Acacia trees, 29
acetylcholine, 159
adrenaline, 17, 101–2, 266
African violets, 189
allergies, 170–2, 176, 220, 227–8
  anti-allergenic compounds, 267
Alzheimer's disease, 166, 181
ambergris, 84
American basswood (*Tilia
  americana*), 42
American beech (*Fagus
  grandifolia*), 42
American sweet gum (*Liquidambar
  styraciflua*), 227
amino acids, 165
ammonia, 87
Amomum spp., 85
amylase, 129, 201, 224–5
Andrews, Matthew, and Birgitta
  Gatersleben, 218–19
Andrianandrasana, Herizo, 62
anthocyanin, 56–7, 72
Anthurium spp., 189
antibiotics, 165–6, 168, 179
antidepressants, 10, 18, 229
apoptosis, 100

Appalachian forests, 80
Appleton, John, 219
araucaria, 27, 147
Araucariaceae family, 200
Aristotle, 85–6, 158
arrowhead plant (*Syngonium
  podophyllum*), 195
Art Nouveau, 190
asthma, 105, 171, 185, 193, 228, 267
Attention Deficit Hyperactivity
  Disorder, 143
Attention Restoration Theory,
  23–5, 202
autism, 143, 166, 181
autoimmune responses and
  diseases, 163, 170–1, 178,
  181–2, 267
auxin, 52, 56

baby rubberplant (*Peperomia
  obtusifolia*), 195
Balling, John, and Falk, John, 30–1
Barton, Jo, and Pretty, Jules, 243–4
base notes, 84
begonia (*Begonia pavonia*), 46
benzodiazepines, 108
beta-blockers, 18
betalains, 69–70

About the Author

Kathy Willis CBE is professor of biodiversity in the department of biology and the principal of St Edmund Hall, University of Oxford. She is also a crossbench peer in the House of Lords. Previous roles include director of science at the Royal Botanic Gardens, Kew, and a member of the UK Government's Natural Capital Committee. She has extensive broadcast experience and, in 2015, Kathy was awarded the Michael Faraday Medal for public communication of science from the Royal Society.

A Note on the Type

The text of this book is set in Bembo, which was first used in 1495 by the Venetian printer Aldus Manutius for Cardinal Bembo's *De Aetna*. The original types were cut for Manutius by Francesco Griffo. Bembo was one of the types used by Claude Garamond (1480–1561) as a model for his Romain de l'Université, and so it was a forerunner of what became the standard European type for the following two centuries. Its modern form follows the original types and was designed for Monotype in 1929.